Teen Health Series

Skin Health Information
For Teens, Fourth Edition

Skin Health Information
For Teens, Fourth Edition

Health Tips About Dermatological Disorders
And Activities That Affect The Skin, Hair, And Nails

Including Facts About Acne, Infectious Skin Conditions,
Skin Cancer, Skin Injuries, And Other Conditions And
Lifestyle Choices, Such As Tanning, Tattooing, And Piercing

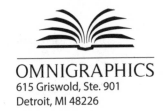

OMNIGRAPHICS
615 Griswold, Ste. 901
Detroit, MI 48226

Bibliographic Note
Because this page cannot legibly accommodate all the copyright notices, the Bibliographic Note portion of the Preface constitutes an extension of the copyright notice.

* * *

OMNIGRAPHICS
Siva Ganesh Maharaja, *Managing Editor*

* * *

Copyright © 2018 Omnigraphics
ISBN 978-0-7808-1579-7
E-ISBN 978-0-7808-1580-3

Library of Congress Cataloging-in-Publication Data

Names: Omnigraphics, Inc., issuing body.

Title: Skin health information for teens: health tips about dermatological disorders and activities that affect the skin, hair, and nails including facts about acne, infectious skin conditions, skin cancer, skin injuries, and other conditions and lifestyle choices, such as tanning, tattooing, and piercing.

Description: Fourth edition. | Detroit, MI: Omnigraphics, Inc., [2017] | Series: Teen health series | Audience: Grade 9 to 12. | Includes bibliographical references and index.

Identifiers: LCCN 2017033342 (print) | LCCN 2017033530 (ebook) | ISBN 9780780815803 (eBook) | ISBN 9780780815797 (hardcover: alk. paper)

Subjects: LCSH: Teenagers--Health and hygiene. | Skin--Care and hygiene. | Beauty, Personal.

Classification: LCC RA777 (ebook) | LCC RA777.S546 2017 (print) | DDC 646.7/208352--dc23

LC record available at https://lccn.loc.gov/2017033342

Table Of Contents

Part Four: Other Diseases And Disorders Affecting The Skin

Part Five: Skin Injuries

Part Six: Taking Care Of Your Skin, Hair, And Nails

Part Seven: If You Need More Information

Preface

About This Book

From the thinnest layer of skin on the eyelids to the thickest layer on the soles of the feet, skin protects the entire body and is essential to survival. But skin itself is vulnerable to rashes, infections, injuries, and disease, from the relatively minor to the extremely serious. Coping with diseases like skin cancer and scleroderma can leave teens overwhelmed and desperate for information. And while conditions like acne and vitiligo are not physically threatening, they can be emotionally devastating at a period when appearance is all-important. Other conditions that might seem harmless—like birthmarks, blushing, and excess sweating—also can affect selfesteem. In addition, teens make choices about sun and outdoor exposure, body art, and beauty products that have the potential to damage the skin's health and weaken its protective ability.

Skin Health Information For Teens, Fourth Edition provides updated information on medical conditions that affect the skin, hair, and nails. It describes the basics of healthy skin and skin care, taking different skin types into account. It explains prevention, warning signs, and treatment options for skin cancer and spells out the risks of tanning—outside and indoors. Acne is discussed in depth, including scar treatment and developing a healthy self-image even with facial skin that is "different." Care of common conditions—such as allergic rashes, viral infections like cold sores, and injuries like cuts, scrapes, bruises, bites, and stings—is also covered. Information to help teens make healthy choices as they express themselves through cosmetics, piercing, and tattoos is also included. Finally, the book provides a section on further reading about skin concerns and a directory of additional resources.

How To Use This Book

This book is divided into parts and chapters. Parts focus on broad areas of interest; chapters are devoted to single topics within a part.

Part One: Skin Basics provides information about skin anatomy and the skin's protective function. It discusses why freckles and brown spots occur and how teens blush. It includes information on ethnicity and specific skin conditions. The effects of smoking on looks are described.

Part Two: Acne focuses on the causes of acne and how it develops in teens. It details treatments such as over-the-counter products, prescription medicines, and dermatologic procedures for treating acne scars. The psychological effects of acne are discussed.

Part Three: Infectious Conditions Of The Skin describes bacterial, viral, fungal, and parasitic diseases that affect the skin. Bacterial concerns include impetigo and necrotizing fasciitis, the so-called flesh-eating disease. The viral conditions addressed include cold sores, warts, and human papillomavirus (HPV). Chapters related to fungal and parasitic infections discuss ringworm, athlete's foot, Lyme disease, scabies, and others.

Part Four: Other Disorders And Diseases Affecting The Skin discusses a variety of inherited, allergic, autoimmune, and other skin disorders. It explains conditions that are medically benign but cause for concern in self-conscious teens, such as cellulite, stretch marks, vitiligo, rosacea, and hyperhidrosis (excessive sweating). It also describes itching, hives, eczema, lupus, scleroderma, psoriasis, and moles. Skin cancer—particularly melanoma and basal cell carcinoma—is detailed, including causes, detection, diagnosis, treatment, and prevention.

Part Five: Skin Injuries provides facts about prevention, first aid, and treatment of scrapes, cuts, bruises, insect bites and stings, animal bites, poison ivy and poison oak, and frostbite. It covers care of scars and scar removal, corns and calluses, and nail abnormalities. Burn assessment and treatment are explained, along with a section on prevention of burn injuries in teen workers. Skin picking is described and coping mechanisms are suggested.

Part Six: Taking Care Of Your Skin, Hair, And Nails describes self-care and lifestyle choices teens make that affect their appearance and health. It details concerns about outdoor and indoor tanning and offers facts about tanning alternatives. Safety precautions are given for teens interested in tattoos or piercing. Hair health, including damage from hair-care products, and hair loss are discussed. Nail care and abnormalities are also addressed.

Part Seven: If You Need More Information provides suggestions for additional reading on topics related to skin and a list of further resources.

Bibliographic Note

This volume contains documents and excerpts from publications issued by the following government agencies: Centers for Disease Control and Prevention (CDC); Genetic and Rare Diseases Information Center (GARD); Genetics Home Reference (GHR); Health Resources and Services Administration (HRSA); National Cancer Institute (NCI); National Institute of Arthritis and Musculoskeletal and Skin Diseases (NIAMS); National Institute of General

Medical Sciences (NIGMS); National Institutes of Health (NIH); *NIH News in Health*; Office on Women's Health (OWH); U.S. Department of Agriculture (USDA); U.S. Department of Health and Human Services (HHS); and U.S. Food and Drug Administration (FDA).

It may also contain original material produced by Omnigraphics and reviewed by medical consultants.

The photograph on the front cover is © Margot Pandone/Unsplash.

Medical Review

Omnigraphics contracts with a team of qualified, senior medical professionals who serve as medical consultants for the *Teen Health Series*. As necessary, medical consultants review reprinted and originally written material for currency and accuracy. Citations including the phrase, Reviewed (month, year)" indicate material reviewed by this team. Medical consultation services are provided to the *Teen Health Series* editors by:

Dr. Vijayalakshmi, MBBS, DGO, MD
Dr. Senthil Selvan, MBBS, DCH, MD
Dr. K. Sivanandham, MBBS, DCH, MS (Research), PhD

About The *Teen Health Series*

At the request of librarians serving today's young adults, the *Teen Health Series* was developed as a specially focused set of volumes within Omnigraphics' *Health Reference Series*. Each volume deals comprehensively with a topic selected according to the needs and interests of people in middle school and high school. Teens seeking preventive guidance, information about disease warning signs, medical statistics, and risk factors for health problems will find answers to their questions in the *Teen Health Series*. The *Series*, however, is not intended to serve as a tool for diagnosing illness, in prescribing treatments, or as a substitute for the physician/patient relationship. All people concerned about medical symptoms or the possibility of disease are encouraged to seek professional care from an appropriate healthcare provider.

If there is a topic you would like to see addressed in a future volume of the *Teen Health Series*, please write to:

Editor
Teen Health Series
Omnigraphics
615 Griswold, Ste. 901
Detroit, MI 48226

A Note About Spelling And Style

Teen Health Series editors use *Stedman's Medical Dictionary* as an authority for questions related to the spelling of medical terms and the *Chicago Manual of Style* for questions related to grammatical structures, punctuation, and other editorial concerns. Consistent adherence is not always possible, however, because the individual volumes within the *Series* include many documents from a wide variety of different producers and copyright holders, and the editor's primary goal is to present material from each source as accurately as is possible following the terms specified by each document's producer. This sometimes means that information in different chapters may follow other guidelines and alternate spelling authorities. For example, occasionally a copyright holder may require that eponymous terms be shown in possessive forms (Crohn's disease vs. Crohn disease) or that British spelling norms be retained (leukaemia vs. leukemia).

Part One
Skin Basics

Chapter 1

Why Skin Is So Important

The skin is a vital organ that covers the entire outside of the body, forming a protective barrier against pathogens and injuries from the environment. The skin is the body's largest organ; covering the entire outside of the body, it is about 2 mm thick and weighs approximately six pounds. It shields the body against heat, light, injury, and infection. The skin also helps regulate body temperature, gathers sensory information from the environment, stores water, fat, and vitamin D, and plays a role in the immune system protecting us from disease.

The color, thickness and texture of skin vary over the body. There are two general types of skin; thin and hairy, which is more prevalent on the body, and thick and hairless, which is found on parts of the body that are used heavily and endure a large amount of friction, like the palms of the hands or the soles of the feet.

Basically, the skin is comprised of two layers that cover a third fatty layer. These three layers differ in function, thickness, and strength. The outer layer is called the epidermis; it is a tough protective layer that contains the melanin-producing melanocytes. The second layer (located under the epidermis) is called the dermis; it contains nerve endings, sweat glands, oil glands,

About This Chapter: Text in this chapter begins with excerpts from "Anatomy Of The Skin," Surveillance, Epidemiology and End Results Program (SEER), National Cancer Institute (NCI), December 30, 2016; Text under the heading "Layers Of The Skin" is excerpted from "Layers Of The Skin," Surveillance, Epidemiology and End Results Program (SEER), National Cancer Institute (NCI), July 28, 2017; Text under the heading "Blushing" is © 2018 Omnigraphics. Reviewed August 2017; Text under the heading "Skin Diseases" is excerpted from "Healthy Skin Matters," National Institute of Arthritis and Musculoskeletal and Skin Diseases (NIAMS), October 2015; Text under the heading "Fungal Infections Of The Skin" is excerpted from "Fungal Infections," MedlinePlus, National Institutes of Health (NIH), October 18, 2016; Text under the heading "Hair Basics" is excerpted from "Tips For Healthy Hair," MedlinePlus, National Institutes of Health (NIH), July 6, 2016; Text under the heading "Nails" is excerpted from "Nail Diseases," MedlinePlus, National Institutes of Health (NIH), August 22, 2016; Text under the heading "Scalp And Disorders Of Scalp" is excerpted from "Dandruff, Cradle Cap, And Other Scalp Conditions," MedlinePlus, National Institutes of Health (NIH), October 18, 2016.

and hair follicles. Under these two skin layers is a fatty layer of subcutaneous tissue, known as the subcutis or hypodermis.

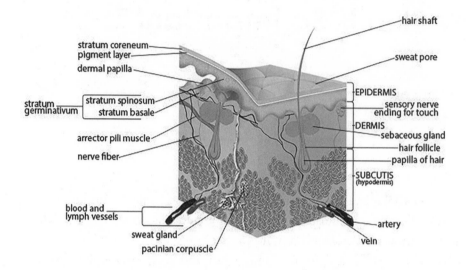

Figure 1.1. Normal Skin

Why Is Healthy Skin Important?

Since your skin plays such an important role in protecting your body, you should keep it as healthy as you can. Th is will help you keep from getting sick or having damage to your bones, muscles, and internal organs.

Your skin also helps keep your body temperature even. If you get too hot, blood vessels near the surface of the skin, called capillaries, enlarge to let the warm blood cool down.

(Source: "Healthy Skin Matters," National Institute of Arthritis and Musculoskeletal and Skin Diseases (NIAMS).)

Layers Of The Skin

The Epidermis

The epidermis is the outermost layer of the skin, and protects the body from the environment. The thickness of the epidermis varies in different types of skin; it is only .05 mm thick on the eyelids, and is 1.5 mm thick on the palms and the soles of the feet. The epidermis contains the melanocytes (the cells in which melanoma develops), the Langerhans' cells (involved in the immune system in the skin), Merkel cells and sensory nerves. The epidermis layer itself is made up of five sublayers that work together to continually rebuild the surface of the skin:

The Basal Cell Layer

The basal layer is the innermost layer of the epidermis, and contains small round cells called basal cells. The basal cells continually divide, and new cells constantly push older ones up toward the surface of the skin, where they are eventually shed. The basal cell layer is also known as the stratum germinativum due to the fact that it is constantly germinating (producing) new cells.

The basal cell layer contains cells called melanocytes. Melanocytes produce the skin coloring or pigment known as melanin, which gives skin its tan or brown color and helps protect the deeper layers of the skin from the harmful effects of the sun. Sun exposure causes melanocytes to increase production of melanin in order to protect the skin from damaging ultraviolet rays, producing a suntan. Patches of melanin in the skin cause birthmarks, freckles and age spots. Melanoma develops when melanocytes undergo malignant transformation.

Merkel cells, which are tactile cells of neuroectodermal origin, are also located in the basal layer of the epidermis.

The Squamous Cell Layer

The squamous cell layer is located above the basal layer, and is also known as the stratum spinosum or "spiny layer" due to the fact that the cells are held together with spiny projections. Within this layer are the basal cells that have been pushed upward, however these maturing cells are now called squamous cells, or keratinocytes. Keratinocytes produce keratin, a tough, protective protein that makes up the majority of the structure of the skin, hair, and nails.

The squamous cell layer is the thickest layer of the epidermis, and is involved in the transfer of certain substances in and out of the body. The squamous cell layer also contains cells called Langerhans cells. These cells attach themselves to antigens that invade damaged skin and alert the immune system to their presence.

The Stratum Granulosum And The Stratum Lucidum

The keratinocytes from the squamous layer are then pushed up through two thin epidermal layers called the stratum granulosum and the stratum lucidum. As these cells move further towards the surface of the skin, they get bigger and flatter and adhere together, and then eventually become dehydrated and die. This process results in the cells fusing together into layers of tough, durable material, which continue to migrate up to the surface of the skin.

The Stratum Corneum

The stratum corneum is the outermost layer of the epidermis, and is made up of 10 to 30 thin layers of continually shedding, dead keratinocytes. The stratum corneum is also known as the "horny layer," because its cells are toughened like an animal's horn. As the outermost cells age and wear down, they are replaced by new layers of strong, long-wearing cells. The stratum corneum is sloughed off continually as new cells take its place, but this shedding process slows down with age. Complete cell turnover occurs every 28 to 30 days in young adults.

The Dermis

The dermis is located beneath the epidermis and is the thickest of the three layers of the skin (1.5 to 4 mm thick), making up approximately 90 percent of the thickness of the skin. The main functions of the dermis are to regulate temperature and to supply the epidermis with nutrient-saturated blood. Much of the body's water supply is stored within the dermis. This layer contains most of the skins' specialized cells and structures, including:

- **Blood Vessels:** The blood vessels supply nutrients and oxygen to the skin and take away cell waste and cell products. The blood vessels also transport the vitamin D produced in the skin back to the rest of the body.

- **Lymph Vessels:** The lymph vessels bathe the tissues of the skin with lymph, a milky substance that contains the infection-fighting cells of the immune system. These cells work to destroy any infection or invading organisms as the lymph circulates to the lymph nodes.

- **Hair Follicles:** The hair follicle is a tube-shaped sheath that surrounds the part of the hair that is under the skin and nourishes the hair.

- **Sweat Glands:** The average person has about 3 million sweat glands. Sweat glands are classified according to two types:

  - Apocrine glands are specialized sweat glands that can be found only in the armpits and pubic region. These glands secrete a milky sweat that encourages the growth of the bacteria responsible for body odor.

  - Eccrine glands are the true sweat glands. Found over the entire body, these glands regulate body temperature by bringing water via the pores to the surface of the skin, where it evaporates and reduces skin temperature. These glands can produce up to two liters of sweat an hour, however, they secrete mostly water, which doesn't encourage the growth of odor-producing bacteria.

- **Sebaceous glands:** Sebaceous, or oil, glands, are attached to hair follicles and can be found everywhere on the body except for the palms of the hands and the soles of the feet. These glands secrete oil that helps keep the skin smooth and supple. The oil also helps keep skin waterproof and protects against an overgrowth of bacteria and fungi on the skin.

- **Nerve Endings:** The dermis layer also contains pain and touch receptors that transmit sensations of pain, itch, pressure and information regarding temperature to the brain for interpretation. If necessary, shivering (involuntary contraction and relaxation of muscles) is triggered, generating body heat.

- **Collagen and Elastin:** The dermis is held together by a protein called collagen, made by fibroblasts. Fibroblasts are skin cells that give the skin its strength and resilience. Collagen is a tough, insoluble protein found throughout the body in the connective tissues that hold muscles and organs in place. In the skin, collagen supports the epidermis, lending it its durability. Elastin, a similar protein, is the substance that allows the skin to spring back into place when stretched and keeps the skin flexible.

The dermis layer is made up of two sublayers:

The Papillary Layer

The upper, papillary layer, contains a thin arrangement of collagen fibers. The papillary layer supplies nutrients to select layers of the epidermis and regulates temperature. Both of these functions are accomplished with a thin, extensive vascular system that operates similarly to other vascular systems in the body. Constriction and expansion control the amount of blood that flows through the skin and dictate whether body heat is dispelled when the skin is hot or conserved when it is cold.

The Reticular Layer

The lower, reticular layer, is thicker and made of thick collagen fibers that are arranged in parallel to the surface of the skin. The reticular layer is denser than the papillary dermis, and it strengthens the skin, providing structure and elasticity. It also supports other components of the skin, such as hair follicles, sweat glands, and sebaceous glands.

The Subcutis

The subcutis is the innermost layer of the skin, and consists of a network of fat and collagen cells. The subcutis is also known as the hypodermis or subcutaneous layer, and functions as both an insulator, conserving the body's heat, and as a shock-absorber, protecting the inner organs. It also stores fat as an energy reserve for the body. The blood vessels, nerves, lymph vessels, and hair follicles also cross through this layer. The thickness of the subcutis layer varies throughout the body and from person to person.

Blushing[1]

Blushing is an involuntary reaction that causes a person's face to redden due to any embarrassment or stress. Physiologically, the same mechanism that is responsible for the bodily "fight or flight" response causes blushing. When a person encounters sudden or strong emotions, the sympathetic nervous system responds by widening the blood vessels in the face. The sudden rushing of blood in the face causes the redness associated with blushing.

It takes a minute or two for facial blushing to disappear and it can be a source of embarrassment. Frequent blushing in some individuals can be a hindrance in personal and professional life.

In addition to the emotional triggers, hot and spicy foods, hot drinks, increased physical activity, sudden increase or decrease in temperature, fever, certain medical conditions, and medications can cause blushing.

Blushing can be treated with cognitive behavioral therapy and medications.

[1]Reference

"Blushing," NHS Choices, October 3, 2016.

Skin Diseases

There are many diseases that can affect your skin. Some like vitiligo cause the skin to lose its natural color, and some like alopecia areata can make the hair fall out. Another skin disease like epidermolysis bullosa can cause painful blisters. Psoriasis can cause itchy, scaly red patches. Go see your doctor if you think you might have a skin disease.

Fungal Infections Of The Skin

If you have ever had athlete's foot or a yeast infection, you can blame a fungus. A fungus is a primitive organism. Mushrooms, mold and mildew are examples. Fungi live in air, in soil, on plants and in water. Some live in the human body. Only about half of all types of fungi are harmful.

Some fungi reproduce through tiny spores in the air. You can inhale the spores or they can land on you. As a result, fungal infections often start in the lungs or on the skin. You are more likely to get a fungal infection if you have a weakened immune system or take antibiotics.

Fungi can be difficult to kill. For skin and nail infections, you can apply medicine directly to the infected area. Oral antifungal medicines are also available for serious infections.

Hair Basics

The average person has 5 million hairs. Hair grows all over your body except on your lips, palms, and the soles of your feet. It takes about a month for healthy hair to grow half an inch. Most hairs grow for up to six years and then fall out. New hairs grow in their place.

Hair helps keep you warm. It also protects your eyes, ears, and nose from small particles in the air.

Nails

Your toenails and fingernails protect the tissues of your toes and fingers. They are made up of layers of a hardened protein called keratin, which is also in your hair and skin. The health of your nails can be a clue to your overall health. Healthy nails are usually smooth and consistent in color. Specific types of nail discoloration and changes in growth rate can be signs of lung, heart, kidney, and liver diseases, as well as diabetes and anemia. White spots and vertical ridges are harmless.

Nail problems that sometimes require treatment include:

- Bacterial and fungal infections
- Ingrown nails
- Tumors
- Warts

Keeping your nails clean, dry, and trimmed can help you avoid some problems. Do not remove the cuticle, which can cause infection.

Scalp And Disorders Of Scalp

Your scalp is the skin on the top of your head. Unless you have hair loss, hair grows on your scalp. Different skin problems can affect your scalp.

Dandruff is a flaking of the skin. The flakes are yellow or white. Dandruff may make your scalp feel itchy. It usually starts after puberty, and is more common in men. Dandruff is usually a symptom of seborrheic dermatitis, or seborrhea. It is a skin condition that can also cause redness and irritation of the skin.

Most of the time, using a dandruff shampoo can help control your dandruff. If that does not work, contact your healthcare provider.

There is a type of seborrheic dermatitis that babies can get. It is called cradle cap. It usually lasts a few months, and then goes away on its own. Besides the scalp, it can sometimes affect other parts of the body, such as the eyelids, armpits, groin, and ears. Normally, washing your baby's hair every day with a mild shampoo and gently rubbing their scalp with your fingers or a soft brush can help. For severe cases, your healthcare provider may give you a prescription shampoo or cream to use.

Other problems that can affect the scalp include:

- **Scalp ringworm**, a fungal infection that causes itchy, red patches on your head. It can also leave bald spots. It usually affects children.

- **Scalp psoriasis**, which causes itchy or sore patches of thick, red skin with silvery scales. About half of the people with psoriasis have it on their scalp.

Chapter 2

Freckles And Brown Spots

Freckles

The medical term for freckle is "ephilis." Freckles are small, flat, brown spots that can appear anywhere on the body, but are seen mostly on the face and other sun-exposed areas of the skin. They are common among children and light-skinned people, especially people with red hair, but they can appear on those with dark skin as darker brown spots. Freckles are caused by the localized buildup of skin pigment in skin cells. Melanin (skin pigment) is made up of cells known as melanocytes. When exposed to the sun, melanocytes produce more melanin and that melanin spreads over surrounding skin cells called keratinocytes. Accumulated melanin in keratinocytes gives color to ephilides (freckles). Freckles usually fade away during winter as the skin cells with more melanin are replaced by new ones. Freckles generally diminish with age.

Causes Of Freckles

The tendency to freckle is considered an inherited trait. In rare cases genetic diseases such as Xeroderma pigmentosum can cause freckles.

Treatment For Freckles

Freckles are harmless, benign (noncancercous) condition, so there is no need to treat them. You can help prevent freckling by using sunscreen covering your skin and wearing a brimmed hat while in the sun. Light-skinned people who tend to freckle easily are also at greater risk

"Freckles And Brown Spots," © 2018 Omnigraphics. Reviewed August 2017.

for skin cancer. Less exposure to the sun and using sunscreens could help reduce the risk of skin cancer.

Lentigines

Lentigines are large, flat, brown spots on the face, arms, and legs that result from buildup of melanocytes. They are mainly caused by exposure to the sun, but can also occur after some medical procedures. The spots usually occur during middle age and are also known as liver spots or age spots. Unlike freckles, lentigines stay for longer periods of time and do not fade away in winter. Lentigines are common among light-skinned people.

Treatment For Lentigines

A doctor will identify lentigines through a physical examination. It is important to distinguish early on if a spot is a harmless lentigo or a cancerous melanoma. If a large spot has recently surfaced, has irregular borders, is made up of two or three colors then a biopsy should be performed. Lentigines, however, are harmless and do not need medical treatment. However, some people dislike their appearance and can have their spots cosmetically treated using laser surgery, skin creams such as retinoids or bleaching agents, or cryotherapy (a method of freezing).

Brown Marks

Brown marks other than freckles or lentigines can be of different shapes and texture. If the mark contains a high amount of keratinocytes (skin cells), it can become scaly. These marks may be either actinic keratoses (damage by sun) or seborrhoeic keratoses (senile warts). Certain pigmentations on the face could also be because of a chronic disorder called melasma.

Treatment For Brown Marks

Brown marks can be treated in a number of ways, including antiaging creams, cryotherapy, chemical peels, and laser surgery.

Prevention Of Brown Marks

The best way to prevent brown marks is to protect oneself from the sun light. Sunscreens (SPF 50+) and protective clothing can also help prevent the brown marks.

References

1. "Brown Spots And Freckles," DermNet New Zealand, n.d.

2. "Moles, Freckles, Skin Tags, Lentigines, & Seborrheic Keratoses," Cleveland Clinic, n.d.

3. "What Is The Difference Between Age Spots, Sun Spots And Freckles?" Asherah Health, September 20, 2015.

Chapter 3

Ethnicity And Skin

Pigmentation means coloring. Skin pigmentation disorders affect the color of your skin. Your skin gets its color from a pigment called melanin. Special cells in the skin make melanin. When these cells become damaged or unhealthy, it affects melanin production. Some pigmentation disorders affect just patches of skin. Others affect your entire body.

If your body makes too much melanin, your skin gets darker. Pregnancy, Addison disease, and sun exposure all can make your skin darker. If your body makes too little melanin, your skin gets lighter. Vitiligo is a condition that causes patches of light skin. Albinism is a genetic condition affecting a person's skin. A person with albinism may have no color, lighter than normal skin color, or patchy missing skin color. Infections, blisters and burns can also cause lighter skin. Postinflammatory hyperpigmentation (PIH) and rosacea are skin conditions that usually affect ethnic skin.

Postinflammatory Hyperpigmentation (PIH)

Postinflammatory hyperpigmentation (PIH) is an acquired hypermelanosis that occurs after cutaneous inflammation or injury. This process can occur in all skin types but more frequently affects darker skinned patients, such as African-Americans, Hispanics,

About This Chapter: Text in this chapter begins with excerpts from "Skin Pigmentation Disorders," MedlinePlus, National Institutes of Health (NIH), May 2, 2016; Text under the heading "Postinflammatory Hyperpigmentation (PIH)" is excerpted from "An In Vivo Model For Postinflammatory Hyperpigmentation," ClinicalTrials.gov, National Institutes of Health (NIH), February 22, 2017; Text under the heading "Rosacea" is excerpted from "Red In The Face," NIH News in Health, National Institutes of Health (NIH), August 2012. Reviewed August 2017; Text under the heading "Skin Care And Sun Protection For Ethnic Skin Types" is excerpted from "Sun And Skin," NIH News in Health, National Institutes of Health (NIH), July 2014.

Asians, Native Americans, Pacific Islanders, and those of Middle Eastern descent. PIH can occur after infection, allergic reactions, contact dermatitis, some medications, burn, following procedures, or inflammatory disease such as acne. In skin of color, PIH frequently occurs in resolving acne lesions and can persist for months after the acne lesion itself has disappeared. In many cases, the resulting PIH can be more distressing than the original insult.

Rosacea

Some people think of a rosy complexion as a sign of good health. But red patches on the face may point to something more troubling—a long-lasting skin disorder called rosacea.

Rosacea may start as redness on the cheeks, nose, chin, or forehead. It might even look like an outbreak of pimples. But over time, the condition can worsen. Inflammation can make affected skin swollen and sensitive. Red, thick, bumpy skin may appear on the face, causing discomfort and distress. Up to half of people with rosacea also develop eye problems. Eyelids may become inflamed, and vision impaired. Rosacea affects an estimated 14 million Americans. The causes of rosacea are unclear. The condition tends to run in families, so genes likely play a role.

Although anyone can get rosacea, lighter-skinned populations are at greater risk. People who blush frequently may also be more vulnerable. Women are 3 to 4 times more likely than men to develop rosacea. But rosacea symptoms are generally more severe in men. Rosacea symptoms can come and go, flaring up for weeks or months and then subsiding. Over time, the facial redness can deepen and become more permanent.

Things that cause flare-ups are called triggers. Although they vary from person to person, common triggers include hot foods or beverages, spicy foods, alcohol, extreme temperatures, sunlight, stress, exercise, and hot baths.

Because rosacea tends to worsen over time, early detection is critical. There's no test for rosacea, and several other conditions can have similar symptoms. Your doctor needs expertise and experience to make a diagnosis. A dermatologist—a physician who specializes in skin disorders—can aid with rosacea detection and care.

Although there's no cure for rosacea, medical treatments and lifestyle changes can reduce symptoms. Antibiotics taken orally or applied to the skin can lessen redness and bumps. For more serious cases, laser surgery can remove visible blood vessels, reduce redness or correct thickened, bumpy skin.

Skin Care And Sun Protection For Ethnic Skin Types

Sunlight travels to Earth as a mixture of both visible and invisible rays, and waves. Long waves, like radio waves, are harmless to people. But shorter waves, like ultraviolet (UV) light, can cause problems. The longest of these UV rays that reach the Earth's surface are called ultraviolet A (UVA) rays. The shorter ones are called ultraviolet B (UVB) rays.

Too much exposure to UVB rays can lead to sunburn. UVA rays can travel more deeply into the skin than UVB rays, but both can affect your skin's health. When UV rays enter skin cells, they upset delicate processes that affect the skin's growth and appearance. Over time, exposure to these rays can make the skin less elastic. Skin may even become thickened and leathery, wrinkled, or thinned like tissue paper. "The more sun exposure you have, the earlier your skin ages," says Dr. Barnett S. Kramer, a cancer prevention expert at National Institutes of Health (NIH).

Your skin does have ways to prevent or repair such damage. The outermost layer of skin constantly sheds dead skin cells and replaces them. You might have noticed this type of skin repair if you've ever had a bad sunburn. Your skin may peel, but it usually looks normal in a week or two. As you get older, it becomes harder for skin to repair itself. Over time, UV damage can take a toll on your skin and its underlying connective tissue. As a result, your skin may develop more wrinkles and lines.

Too much sun exposure can also raise your risk for skin cancer, the most common type of cancer in the United States. When UV light enters skin cells, it can harm the genetic material called deoxyribonucleic acid (DNA) within. DNA damage can cause changes to cells that make them rapidly grow and divide. This growth can lead to clumps of extra cells called a tumor, or lesion. These may be cancerous (malignant) or harmless (benign). Skin cancer may first appear as a small spot on the skin. Some cancers reach deep into surrounding tissue. They may also spread from the skin to other organs of the body.

"One of the major factors affecting skin health is genetics, which determines the pigment content of your skin. This affects how much protection you have from natural sunlight," explains Katz. Although darker-skinned people have a lower risk for sun-related damage and disease, people of all races and skin color can still get skin cancer.

"Certain genetic mutations contribute to melanoma onset in certain people. You find much less nonmelanoma skin cancer in African Americans, people from the Middle East, or even Asians from the Near East," Katz says.

The best way to protect skin health and prevent skin cancer is to limit sun exposure. Avoid prolonged time in the sun, and choose to be in the shade rather than in direct sunlight. Wear protective clothing and sunglasses, and use sunscreen between 10 a.m. and 4 p.m. Sunscreen is especially important at that time, when the sun rays are most intense.

Sunscreens come labeled with a sun-protection factor (SPF), such as 15, 30, or 50. A sunscreen labeled SPF 15 means it will take you 15 times as long to get a sunburn as it would if you had no sunscreen on. A sunscreen labeled SPF 30 means it would take you 30 times as long to burn.

The effectiveness of sunscreens is affected by several factors. A sunscreen's active ingredients can break down over time, so be sure to check the expiration date on the container. The amount of sunscreen you use and how often you use it affects your protection from the sun. Perspiration and time spent in the water can also reduce sunscreen effectiveness.

> About one-third of U.S. teens aged 14 to 17 years had a sunburn during 2014. About half of non-Hispanic white teens, 22 percent of Hispanic teens, 18 percent of non-Hispanic Asian teens, and 7 percent of non-Hispanic black teens had a sunburn during the past year.
>
> *(Source: "Sun-Protective Behavior Rates," Centers for Disease Control and Prevention (CDC).)*

Some people look to the sun as a source of vitamin D, but it takes just a brief time in the sun to do the trick. "You need very little exposure—something like 10 to 15 minutes a day to the backs of your hands, arms, and face—to get enough," Katz says.

Several factors—like cloudy days or having dark-colored skin—can reduce the amount of vitamin D your skin makes. But you can also get vitamin D from foods or dietary supplements. Check with your healthcare provider about whether you should be taking vitamin D supplements.

Chapter 4

How Smoking Affects The Way You Look

You probably already know that smoking is a huge health risk—and that's reason enough not to light up. But if you want even more inspiration, think about all the things you can do with the money you save if you don't smoke. Also think about how smoking can wreck your good looks. It can turn your teeth and fingers yellow, and can cause wrinkles. Smoking also can make your clothes, breath, and hair smell bad (and you might not notice because you get used to it). Smoking won't make you look cool, either. These days, lots of kids are saying that the really cool thing is to be healthy!

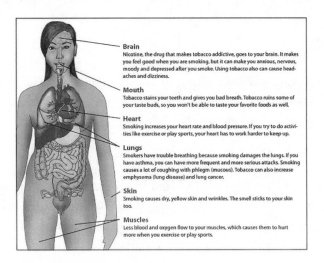

Figure 4.1. How Smoking Affects Your Body

About This Chapter: Text in this chapter begins with excerpts from "Straight Talk About Tobacco," girlshealth. gov, Office on Women's Health (OWH), May 18, 2010. Reviewed August 2017; Text under the heading "Smoking Effects On Parts Of Your Body" is excerpted from "Reasons To Quit—Health Effects," Smokefree.gov, U.S. Department of H██ and Human Services (HHS), June 29, 2016.

Smoking Effects On Parts Of Your Body

Smoking harms nearly every organ of the body. Some of these harmful effects are immediate.

Ears

Hearing loss. Smoking reduces the oxygen supply to the cochlea, a snail-shaped organ in the inner ear. This may result in permanent damage to the cochlea and mild to moderate hearing loss.

Eyes

Blindness and night vision. Smoking causes physical changes in the eyes that can threaten your eyesight. Nicotine from cigarettes restricts the production of a chemical necessary for you to be able to see at night. Also, smoking increases your risk of developing cataracts and macular degeneration (both can lead to blindness).

Mouth

Cavities. Smoking takes a toll on your mouth. Smokers have more oral health problems than nonsmokers, like mouth sores, ulcers, and gum disease. You are more likely to have cavities and lose your teeth at a younger age. You are also more likely to get cancers of the mouth and throat.

Face

Smoker's face. Smoking can cause your skin to be dry and lose elasticity, leading to wrinkles and stretch marks. Your skin tone may become dull and grayish. By your early 30s, wrinkles can begin to appear around your mouth and eyes, adding years to your face.

Belly

Bigger belly. Smokers have bigger bellies and less muscle than nonsmokers. They are more likely to develop type 2 diabetes, even if they don't smoke every day. Smoking also makes it harder to control diabetes once you already have it. Diabetes is a serious disease that can lead to blindness, heart disease, kidney failure, and amputations.

Tired Muscles

Muscle deterioration. When you smoke, less blood and oxygen flow to your muscles, making it harder to build muscle. The lack of oxygen also makes muscles tire more easily. Smokers have more muscle aches and pains than nonsmokers.

Benefits Of Quitting

- Quitting smoking at any age has benefits.
- The sooner you quit, the sooner your body can begin to heal.
- Tobacco smoke harms nonsmokers, too.
- Quitting smoking is the single best way to protect your family from secondhand smoke.

(Source: "Smoking And Tobacco Use," Centers for Disease Control and Prevention (CDC).)

Part Two
Acne

Chapter 5

Acne Basics

What Is Acne?[1]

Acne is a disease that affects the skin's oil glands. The small holes in your skin (pores) connect to oil glands under the skin. These glands make an oily substance called sebum. The pores connect to the glands by a canal called a follicle. Inside the follicles, oil carries dead skin cells to the surface of the skin. A thin hair also grows through the follicle and out to the skin. When the follicle of a skin gland clogs up, a pimple grows.

Most pimples are found on the face, neck, back, chest, and shoulders. Acne is not a serious health threat, but it can cause scars.

What Are The Different Types Of Acne Lesions?[2]

- **Comedo (whiteheads or blackheads) or papules.** The comedo is the basic acne lesion, which is a plugged pore. If the plugged pore stays under the skin, it's called a closed comedo and forms a white bump or whitehead. Blackheads are comedos that open up and appear blackish on the surface of the skin. This black color is not due to dirt, but because the air reacts with the excess oil.

This chapter includes text excerpted from documents published by two public domain sources. Text under headings marked 1 are excerpted from "Fast Facts About Acne," National Institute of Arthritis and Musculoskeletal and Skin Diseases (NIAMS), November 2014; Text under headings marked 2 are excerpted from "Acne," Office on Women's Health (OWH), U.S. Department of Health and Human Services (HHS), February 6, 2017.

- **Pustules or pimples.** Pustules or pimples are acne lesions that contain pus and are red at the base.

- **Nodules.** These are more serious acne lesions. They lodge deeper in the skin, are painful, and can cause scarring.

- **Cysts.** Like nodules, these lesions are deep within in the skin, are painful, and are filled with pus, and can cause scarring.

How Does Acne Develop?[1]

Sometimes, the hair, sebum, and skin cells clump together into a plug. The bacteria in the plug cause swelling. Then when the plug starts to break down, a pimple grows.

There are many types of pimples. The most common types are:

- **Whiteheads.** These are pimples that stay under the surface of the skin.

- **Blackheads.** These pimples rise to the skin's surface and look black. The black color is not from dirt.

- **Papules.** These are small pink bumps that can be tender.

- **Pustules.** These pimples are red at the bottom and have pus on top.

- **Nodules.** These are large, painful, solid pimples that are deep in the skin.

- **Cysts.** These deep, painful, pus-filled pimples can cause scars.

Who Gets Acne?[1]

Acne is the most common skin disease. People of all races and ages get acne. But it is most common in teenagers and young adults. An estimated 80 percent of all people between the ages of 11 and 30 have acne outbreaks at some point. Some people in their forties and fifties still get acne.

What Causes Acne?[1]

The cause of acne is unknown. Doctors think certain factors might cause it:

- The hormone increase in teenage years (this can cause the oil glands to plug up more often)

- Hormone changes during pregnancy

- Starting or stopping birth control pills

- Heredity (if your parents had acne, you might get it, too)
- Some types of medicine
- Greasy makeup

Hygiene And Acne[2]

It is a myth that people get acne because they don't wash enough. Too much washing or scrubbing the skin harshly can make acne worse. And washing away surface oils doesn't do much to prevent or cure acne, because it forms under the skin. The best way to clean the face is to gently wash it twice a day with a mild soap or cleanser. Be careful to remove make-up without harsh scrubbing.

Stress And Acne[2]

Stress does not cause acne. But, acne may be a side effect of some medicines used to treat stress or depression. And in some cases, the social and emotional impact of acne lesions causes stress. Talk with your doctor if you have concerns.

Chocolate, Greasy Food, And Acne[2]

While many feel that eating chocolate or greasy foods causes acne, experts have not found a link between the diet and acne. Foods seem to have little effect on acne in most people. But, it's important to eat a healthy diet for good health.

Acne Flare-Ups

The exact cause of acne is unknown, but certain factors can cause it to flare. They include:

- Changing hormone levels in adolescent girls—and adult women 2 to 7 days before their menstrual period starts
- Oil from skin products (moisturizers or cosmetics) or grease in the work environment (for example, a kitchen with fry vats)
- Pressure from sports helmets or equipment, backpacks, tight collars or tight sports uniforms
- Skin irritants, such as pollution and high humidity
- Squeezing or picking at blemishes
- Hard scrubbing of the skin
- Stress

(Source: "Understanding Acne," NIH News in Health, National Institutes of Health (NIH).)

It is a myth that women get acne because they don't wash enough. Too much washing or scrubbing the skin harshly can make acne worse. And washing away surface oils doesn't do much to prevent or cure acne, because it forms under the skin. The best way to clean the face is to gently wash it twice a day with a mild soap or cleanser. Be careful to remove make-up without harsh scrubbing.

How Is Acne Treated?[1]

Acne is treated by doctors who work with skin problems (dermatologists). Treatment tries to:

- Heal pimples

- Stop new pimples from forming

- Prevent scarring

- Help reduce the embarrassment of having acne

Early treatment is the best way to prevent scars. Your doctor may suggest over-the-counter (OTC) or prescription drugs. Some acne medicines are put right on the skin. Other medicines are pills that you swallow. The doctor may tell you to use more than one medicine.

Birthcontrol Pills And Acne Treatment[2]

For women who break out mainly around their menstrual cycle, some birth control pills can help. Research shows that these pills can clear acne by slowing down overactive oil glands in the skin. Sometimes, birth control pills are used along with a drug called spironolactone to treat acne in adult females. This medication lowers levels of the hormone androgen in the body. Androgen stimulates the skin's oil glands. Side effects of this drug include irregular menstruation, breast tenderness, headache and fatigue. Spironolactone is not appropriate therapy for all patients.

How Should People With Acne Care For Their Skin?[1]

Here are some ways to care for skin if you have acne:

- **Clean skin gently.** Use a mild cleanser in the morning, evening, and after heavy workouts. Scrubbing the skin does not stop acne. It can even make the problem worse.

- **Try not to touch your skin.** People who squeeze, pinch, or pick their pimples can get scars or dark spots on their skin.

- **Shave carefully.** If you shave, you can try both electric and safety razors to see which works best. With safety razors, use a sharp blade. Also, it helps to soften your beard with soap and water before putting on shaving cream. Shave lightly and only when you have to.

- **Stay out of the sun.** Many acne medicines can make people more likely to sunburn. Being in the sun a lot can also make skin wrinkle and raise the risk of skin cancer.

- **Choose makeup carefully.** All makeup should be oil free. Look for the word "noncomedogenic" on the label. This means that the makeup will not clog up your pores. But some people still get acne even if they use these products.

- **Shampoo your hair regularly.** If your hair is oily, you may want to shampoo daily.

What Things Can Make Acne Worse?[1]

Some things can make acne worse:

- Changing hormone levels in teenage girls and adult women 2 to 7 days before their period starts

- Pressure from bike helmets, backpacks, or tight collars

- Pollution and high humidity

- Squeezing or picking at pimples

- Hard scrubbing of the skin.

What Are Some Myths About The Causes Of Acne?[1]

Facts About Acne
- There is no known way to prevent the development of acne.
- Acne is not caused by poor hygiene, sweating, or not washing. While medicated washes containing benzoyl peroxide, resorcinol, salicylic acid, and sulfur are one form of treatment for acne, simple soap and water does not treat the condition.
- Acne is not caused by diet. No scientific connection has been found between diet and acne. No food—not chocolate, fries, pizza, or any other food—has been shown to cause acne.
- Acne does not need to be allowed to run its course.

(Source: "Facing Facts About Acne," U.S. Food and Drug Administration (FDA).)

There are many myths about what causes acne. Dirty skin and stress do not cause acne. Also, chocolate and greasy foods do not cause acne in most people.

Myths About Acne

- Acne is not caused by eating greasy foods like French fries or pizza, or by eating chocolate.
- Scrubbing the skin does not stop acne. It can even make the problem worse. Clean your skin regularly and after heavy workouts. Just remember, don't over scrub.
- Wearing makeup doesn't necessarily cause acne. Choose makeup carefully. All makeup should be oil-free so it doesn't clog up your pores. However, it does help to clean your face regularly to keep makeup from clogging pores, particularly if you are physically active.
- Stress does not cause acne.

(Source: "BAM! Body And Mind—Under The Microscope," Centers for Disease Control and Prevention (CDC).)

Prevent Acne And Acne Scars[2]

You can help prevent acne flare-ups and scars by taking good care of your skin:

- Clean your skin gently with a mild soap or cleanser twice a day — once in the morning and once at night. You should also gently clean the skin after heavy exercise. Avoid strong soaps and rough scrub pads. Harsh scrubbing of the skin may make acne worse. Wash your entire face from under the jaw to the hairline and rinse thoroughly. Remove make-up gently with a mild soap and water. Ask your doctor before using an astringent.

- Wash your hair on a regular basis. If your hair is oily, you may want to wash it more often.

- Do not squeeze or pick at acne lesions. This can cause acne scars.

- Avoid getting sunburned. Many medicines used to treat acne can make you more prone to sunburn. Many people think that the sun helps acne, because the redness from sunburn may make acne lesions less visible. But, too much sun can also increase your risk of skin cancer and early aging of the skin. When you're going to be outside, use sunscreen of at least SPF 15. Also, try to stay in the shade as much as you can.

- Choose make-up and hair care products that are "noncomedogenic" or "nonacnegenic." These products have been made in a way that they don't cause acne. You may also want to use products that are oil-free.

- Avoid things that rub the skin as much as you can, such as backpacks and sports equipment.

- Talk with your doctor about what treatment methods can help your acne. Take your medicines as prescribed. Be sure to tell your doctor if you think medicines you take for other health problems make your acne worse.

Chapter 6

Treating Acne

Acne is often treated by dermatologists, who are doctors who specialize in skin problems. These doctors treat all kinds of acne, particularly severe cases. Doctors who are general or family practitioners, pediatricians, or internists may treat patients with milder cases of acne.

The goals of treatment are to heal existing lesions, stop new lesions from forming, prevent scarring, and minimize the psychological stress and embarrassment caused by this disease. Drug treatment[1] is aimed at reducing several problems that play a part in causing acne:

- abnormal clumping of cells in the follicles

- increased oil production

- bacteria

- inflammation.

[1] *All medicines can have side effects. Some side effects may be more severe than others. You should review the package insert that comes with your medicine and ask your healthcare provider or pharmacist if you have any questions about the possible side effects.*

Depending on the extent of the problem, the doctor may recommend one of several over-the-counter (OTC) medicines and/or prescription medicines. Some of these medicines may be topical (applied to the skin), and others may be oral (taken by mouth). The doctor may suggest using more than one topical medicine or combining oral and topical medicines.

About This Chapter: This chapter includes text excerpted from "Questions And Answers About Acne," National Institute of Arthritis and Musculoskeletal and Skin Diseases (NIAMS), September 2016.

Treatment For Blackheads, Whiteheads, And Mild Inflammatory Acne

Doctors usually recommend an OTC or prescription topical medicine for people with mild signs of acne. Topical medicine is applied directly to the acne lesions or to the entire area of affected skin.

There are several OTC topical medicines used for mild acne. Each works a little differently. Following are some of the most common ones:

- **Benzoyl peroxide.** Kills *Propionibacterium acnes (P. acnes)*, and may also reduce oil production
- **Resorcinol.** Can help break down blackheads and whiteheads
- **Salicylic acid.** Helps break down blackheads and whiteheads. Also helps cut down the shedding of cells lining the hair follicles
- **Sulfur.** Helps break down blackheads and whiteheads.

Topical OTC medicines are available in many forms, such as gels, lotions, creams, soaps, or pads. In some people, OTC acne medicines may cause side effects such as skin irritation, burning, or redness, which often get better or go away with continued use of the medicine. If you experience severe or prolonged side effects, you should report them to your doctor.

OTC topical medicines are somewhat effective in treating acne when used regularly; however, it may take up to 8 weeks before you see noticeable improvement.

Treatment For Moderate-To-Severe Inflammatory Acne

People with moderate-to-severe inflammatory acne may be treated with prescription topical or oral medicines, alone or in combination.

Prescription Topical Medicines

Several types of prescription topical medicines are used to treat acne. They include:

- **Antibiotics.** Help stop or slow the growth of bacteria and reduce inflammation
- **Vitamin A derivatives (retinoids).** Unplug existing comedones (plural of comedo), allowing other topical medicines, such as antibiotics, to enter the follicles. Some may

also help decrease the formation of comedones. These drugs contain an altered form of vitamin A. Some mild forms of retinoids are available without a prescription.

- **Others.** May destroy *Propionibacterium acnes* (*P. acnes*) and reduce oil production or help stop or slow the growth of bacteria and reduce inflammation.

Like OTC topical medicines, prescription topical medicines come as creams, lotions, solutions, gels, or pads. Your doctor will consider your skin type when prescribing a product. Creams and lotions provide moisture and tend to be good choices for people with sensitive skin. If you have very oily skin or live in a hot, humid climate, you may prefer an alcohol-based gel or solution, which tends to dry the skin. Your doctor will tell you how to apply the medicine and how often to use it.

For some people, prescription topical medicines cause minor side effects including stinging, burning, redness, peeling, scaling, or discoloration of the skin. With some medicines, these side effects usually decrease or go away after the medicine is used for a period of time. If side effects are severe or don't go away, notify your doctor.

Prescription Oral Medicines

For patients with moderate-to-severe acne, doctors often prescribe oral antibiotics. Oral antibiotics are thought to help control acne by curbing the growth of bacteria and reducing inflammation. Prescription oral and topical medicines may be combined. Common antibiotics used to treat acne are tetracycline, minocycline, and doxycycline.

Other oral medicines less commonly used are clindamycin, erythromycin, or sulfonamides. Some people taking these antibiotics have side effects, such as an upset stomach, dizziness or lightheadedness, changes in skin color, and increased tendency to sunburn. Because tetracyclines may affect tooth and bone formation in fetuses and young children, these drugs are not given to pregnant women or children under age 14. There is some concern, although it has not been proven, that tetracycline and minocycline may decrease the effectiveness of birth control pills. Therefore, a backup or another form of birth control may be needed. Prolonged treatment with oral antibiotics may be necessary to achieve the desired results.

Treatment For Severe Nodular Or Cystic Acne

People with nodules or cysts should be treated by a dermatologist. For patients with severe inflammatory acne that does not improve with medicines such as those described above, a doctor may prescribe isotretinoin, a retinoid (vitamin A derivative). Isotretinoin is an oral drug that is usually taken once or twice a day with food for 15 to 20 weeks. It markedly reduces the size of the oil glands so that much less oil is produced. As a result, the growth of bacteria is decreased.

Advantages Of Isotretinoin

Isotretinoin is a very effective medicine that can help prevent scarring. After 15 to 20 weeks of treatment with isotretinoin, acne completely or almost completely goes away in most patients. In those patients where acne recurs after a course of isotretinoin, the doctor may institute another course of the same treatment or prescribe other medicines.

Disadvantages Of Isotretinoin

Isotretinoin can cause birth defects in the developing fetus of a pregnant woman. **It is important that women of childbearing age are not pregnant and do not get pregnant while taking this medicine.** Women must use two separate effective forms of birth control at the same time for 1 month before treatment begins, during the entire course of treatment, and for 1 full month after stopping the drug. You should ask your doctor when it is safe to get pregnant after you have stopped taking isotretinoin.

Some people with acne become depressed by the changes in the appearance of their skin. Changes in mood may be intensified during treatment or soon after completing a course of medicines like isotretinoin. There have been a number of reported suicides and suicide attempts in people taking isotretinoin; however, the connection between isotretinoin and suicide or depression is not known. Nevertheless, if you or someone you know feels unusually sad or has other symptoms of depression, such as loss of appetite, loss of interest in once-loved activities, or trouble concentrating, it's important to consult your doctor.

Talk to your doctor or pharmacist about the side effects of isotretinoin. To determine if isotretinoin should be stopped if side effects occur, your doctor may test your blood before you start treatment and periodically during treatment. Side effects usually go away after the medicine is stopped.

Other Treatments For Acne

Doctors may use other types of procedures in addition to drug therapy to treat patients with acne. For example, the doctor may remove the patient's comedones during office visits. Sometimes the doctor will inject corticosteroids directly into lesions to help reduce the size and pain of inflamed cysts and nodules.

Early treatment is the best way to prevent acne scars. Once scarring has occurred, the doctor may suggest a medical or surgical procedure to help reduce the scars. A superficial laser may be used to treat irregular scars. Dermabrasion (or microdermabrasion), which is a form of "sanding down" scars, is sometimes used. Another treatment option for deep scars caused by cystic acne is the transfer of fat from another part of the body to the scar. A doctor may also inject a synthetic filling material under the scar to improve its appearance.

Chapter 7

Isotretinoin Warning

What Is Accutane (Isotretinoin)?

Accutane (Isotretinoin) is a medicine taken by mouth to treat the most severe form of acne (nodular acne) that cannot be cleared up by any other acne treatments, including antibiotics. Accutane can cause serious side effects. Accutane can only be:

- prescribed by doctors that are registered in the iPLEDGE program

- dispensed by a pharmacy that is registered with the iPLEDGE program

- given to patients who are registered in the iPLEDGE program and agree to do everything required in the program

> U.S. Food and Drug Administration (FDA) has approved a strengthened risk management program called iPLEDGE, to minimize fetal exposure to Accutane (isotretinoin) and its generic equivalents.

What Is Severe Nodular Acne?

Severe nodular acne is when many red, swollen, tender lumps form in the skin. These can be the size of pencil erasers or larger. If untreated, nodular acne can lead to permanent scars.

About This Chapter: Text beginning with the heading "What Is Accutane (Isotretinoin)?" is excerpted from "Accutane Medication Guide," U.S. Food and Drug Administration (FDA), January 2010. Reviewed August 2017; Text under the heading "FAQs About Isotretinoin And iPLEDGE" is excerpted from "Accutane (Isotretinoin) Questions And Answers," U.S. Food and Drug Administration (FDA), April 30, 2009. Reviewed August 2017.

Who Should Not Take Accutane?

Do not take Accutane if you are pregnant, plan to become pregnant, or become pregnant during Accutane treatment. Accutane causes severe birth defects.

Do not take Accutane if you are allergic to anything in it. Accutane contains parabens as the preservative.

What Should I Tell My Doctor Before Taking Accutane?

Tell your doctor if you or a family member has any of the following health conditions:

- mental problems

- asthma

- liver disease

- diabetes

- heart disease

- bone loss (osteoporosis) or weak bones

- an eating problem called anorexia nervosa (where people eat too little)

- food or medicine allergies

Tell your doctor if you are pregnant or breastfeeding. Accutane must not be used by women who are pregnant or breastfeeding.

Tell your doctor about all of the medicines you take including prescription and nonprescription medicines, vitamins and herbal supplements. Accutane and certain other medicines can interact with each other, sometimes causing serious side effects. Especially tell your doctor if you take:

Vitamin A supplements. Vitamin A in high doses has many of the same side effects as Accutane. Taking both together may increase your chance of getting side effects.

- Tetracycline antibiotics. Tetracycline antibiotics taken with Accutane can increase the chances of getting increased pressure in the brain.

- Progestin-only birth control pills (mini-pills). They may not work while you take Accutane. Ask your doctor or pharmacist if you are not sure what type you are using.

- Dilantin (phenytoin). This medicine taken with Accutane may weaken your bones.

- Corticosteroid medicines. These medicines taken with Accutane may weaken your bones.

- St. John's Wort. This herbal supplement may make birth control pills work less effectively.

These medicines should not be used with Accutane unless your doctor tells you it is okay.

Know the medicines you take. Keep a list of them to show to your doctor and pharmacist. Do not take any new medicine without talking with your doctor.

How Should I Take Accutane?

- You must take Accutane exactly as prescribed. You must also follow all the instructions of the iPLEDGE program. Before prescribing Accutane, your doctor will:

  - explain the iPLEDGE program to you

  - have you sign the Patient Information/Informed Consent (for all patients). Female patients who can get pregnant must also sign another consent form.

You will not be prescribed Accutane if you cannot agree to or follow all the instructions of the iPLEDGE program.

- You will get no more than a 30-day supply of Accutane at a time. This is to make sure you are following the Accutane iPLEDGE program. You should talk with your doctor each month about side effects.

- The amount of Accutane you take has been specially chosen for you. It is based on your body weight, and may change during treatment.

- Take Accutane 2 times a day with a meal, unless your doctor tells you otherwise. Swallow your Accutane capsules whole with a full glass of liquid. Do not chew or suck on the capsule. Accutane can hurt the tube that connects your mouth to your stomach (esophagus) if it is not swallowed whole.

- If you miss a dose, just skip that dose. Do not take 2 doses at the same time.

- If you take too much Accutane or overdose, call your doctor or poison control center right away

- Your acne may get worse when you first start taking Accutane. This should last only a short while. Talk with your doctor if this is a problem for you.

- You must return to your doctor as directed to make sure you don't have signs of serious side effects. Your doctor may do blood tests to check for serious side effects from Accutane. Female patients who can get pregnant will get a pregnancy test each month.

- Female patients who can get pregnant must agree to use 2 separate forms of effective birth control at the same time 1 month before, while taking, and for 1 month after taking Accutane. You must access the iPLEDGE system to answer questions about the program requirements and to enter your 2 chosen forms of birth control. To access the iPLEDGE system, go to www.ipledgeprogram.com or call 1-866-495-0654.

You must talk about effective birth control methods with your doctor or go for a free visit to talk about birth control with another doctor or family planning expert. Your doctor can arrange this free visit, which will be paid for by the company that makes Accutane.

If you have sex at any time without using 2 forms of effective birth control, get pregnant, or miss your expected period, stop using Accutane and call your doctor right away.

What Should I Avoid While Taking Accutane?

- Do not get pregnant while taking Accutane and for 1 month after stopping Accutane.

- Do not breast feed while taking Accutane and for 1 month after stopping Accutane. Researchers do not know if Accutane can pass through your milk and harm the baby.

- Do not give blood while you take Accutane and for 1 month after stopping Accutane. If someone who is pregnant gets your donated blood, her baby may be exposed to Accutane and may be born with birth defects.

- Do not take other medicines or herbal products with Accutane unless you talk to your doctor.

- Do not have cosmetic procedures to smooth your skin, including waxing, dermabrasion, or laser procedures, while you are using Accutane and for at least 6 months after you stop. Accutane can increase your chance of scarring from these procedures. Check with your doctor for advice about when you can have cosmetic procedures.

- Avoid sunlight and ultraviolet lights as much as possible. Tanning machines use ultraviolet lights. Accutane may make your skin more sensitive to light.

- Do not share Accutane with other people. It can cause birth defects and other serious health problems.

What Are The Possible Side Effects Of Accutane?

Skin rash can occur in patients taking Accutane. In some patients a rash can be serious. Stop using Accutane and call your doctor right away if you develop conjunctivitis (red or inflamed eyes, like "pink eye"), a rash with a fever, blisters on legs, arms or face and/or sores in your mouth, throat, nose, eyes, or if your skin begins to peel.

The common, less serious side effects of Accutane are dry skin, chapped lips, dry eyes, and dry nose that may lead to nosebleeds. Call your doctor if you get any side effect that bothers you or that does not go away.

How Should I Store Accutane?

Store Accutane at room temperature, between 59–86°F. Protect from light.

FAQs About Isotretinoin And iPLEDGE

Does iPLEDGE Make It Harder For Patients To Get Isotretinoin?

FDA understands the importance of minimizing any burden imposed upon patients and doctors by iPLEDGE. It is not substantially more difficult for patients to obtain isotretinoin under iPLEDGE than it was for patients who, along with their doctors, were fully compliant with S.M.A.R.T (System to Manage Accutane Related Teratogenicity). It is possible that some doctors and pharmacies will choose not to participate in iPLEDGE. A listing of all registered pharmacies will be available via the internet (www. ipledgeprogram.com) or telephone (1-866-495-0654).

What Happens If A Pharmacy Refuses To Dispense Isotretinoin To A Patient?

There are several reasons why a pharmacy would refuse to dispense isotretinoin to a patient, such as:

- The patient is not registered in iPLEDGE.
- The prescriber is not registered in iPLEDGE.
- The prescription was presented or picked up after the "do not dispense date."
- The pregnancy test results are not in the iPLEDGE system or they are positive.
- The pharmacy is not registered in iPLEDGE.

The patient should talk to the pharmacist or doctor if a pharmacy refuses to dispense isotretinoin for any reason.

If the pharmacy is not registered in iPLEDGE, the patient will be able to access the iPLEDGE program via the internet (www.ipledgeprogram.com) or telephone (1-866-495-0654) for a listing of registered pharmacies.

Chapter 8

Polycystic Ovary Syndrome And Acne

What Is Polycystic Ovary Syndrome (PCOS)

Polycystic ovary syndrome (PCOS) is a common hormone imbalance that affects around 1 out of 10 to 15 women. Girls as young as 11 can get PCOS.

What Are The Signs Of PCOS?

Some common signs of PCOS include:

- Acne

- No periods, irregular periods, or very heavy periods

- Pelvic pain

- Extra hair on your face or other parts of your body, called "hirsutism"

- Weight gain or trouble losing weight

- Patches of dark, thick skin

If you have some of the above signs, you might have PCOS. There may be other reasons that you have one or more of these signs. See a doctor to find out the cause.

About This Chapter: This chapter includes text excerpted from "What Is PCOS?" girlshealth.gov, Office on Women's Health (OWH), April 15, 2014.

What Causes PCOS?

No one knows the exact cause of PCOS. We do know that most of its symptoms come from problems with hormones, or natural body chemicals. Many girls with PCOS have too much insulin, a hormone that helps turn food into energy. Extra insulin can cause the darkened skin you may have on your neck, behind your knees, and other places.

Girls with PCOS also have extra androgens. Although people often think of androgens as male hormones, females have them too. The extra androgen can lead to acne, excess body hair, weight gain, irregular periods, and other PCOS symptoms.

What Tests Are Used To Diagnose PCOS?

If you think you may have PCOS, it's smart to see your doctor. And knowing what to expect during the appointment can make it less stressful. Here's a list of some of what you might experience:

- Questions from your doctor about your menstrual cycle and your health

- Questions about whether other people in your family have similar symptoms

- A physical examination that includes checking your skin and measuring your body mass index (BMI) and waist size

- An examination of your genitals and possibly other parts of your reproductive system

- A blood test to check your hormone levels and blood sugar levels

Does PCOS Mean I Have Cysts On My Ovaries?

The term "polycystic ovaries" means that there are lots of tiny cysts, or little sacs, on the ovaries. Some young women with PCOS have these cysts, but many others do not. Even if you have them, they are not harmful and do not need to be removed.

Will PCOS Affect My Ability To Have Children Someday?

PCOS can cause problems with fertility (ability to get pregnant), but these problems usually can be treated. Treatments include medications to lower your insulin levels and to help you ovulate—or release an egg—each month. If you are concerned about your ability to get pregnant in the future, talk to your doctor.

Does PCOS Put Me At Risk For Other Conditions?

If you have PCOS, you may be at higher risk of other health problems. These include:

- Diabetes

- High cholesterol

- High blood pressure

- Heart disease

- A thickening of the endometrium, or the lining of the uterus, which can eventually lead to cancer if you don't get your period regularly

Getting your PCOS symptoms under control at an early age may help reduce these risks.

What Is The Treatment For PCOS?

There is no cure for PCOS, but there are lots of ways to treat it. You may use a few of them or different ones at different times, depending on your symptoms.

Lifestyle changes are great ways to deal with PCOS. Eating well and staying active are important if you have PCOS. If you are overweight, losing weight may help with symptoms and may reduce health risks related to PCOS. Don't smoke—or try to quit if you've started.

Birth control pills are a very common form of treatment for PCOS. Birth control pills contain hormones that can:

- Correct the PCOS hormone imbalance

- Lower the level of male hormones, which will lessen acne and hair growth

- Regulate your menstrual periods

- Lower the risk of endometrial cancer (which is higher in young women who don't get their periods regularly)

Metformin is another medicine that may help with irregular periods and other PCOS issues. Metformin is sometimes used to help treat diabetes and may help keep your blood sugar closer to normal levels.

Antiandrogens work to reduce the effects of the male hormones on girls with PCOS. They can help clear up acne and hair growth. You can also deal with unwanted hair through electrolysis, hair removal creams, and laser treatment. There are lots of other options for treating acne.

Staying Fit With PCOS

Physical activity can be a great help if you have PCOS. Young women with PCOS often have high levels of the hormone insulin. Having high levels of insulin tells your body to store fat and may contribute to PCOS symptoms. But physical activity can lower your levels of insulin. Any increase in your activity helps, so find a sport or other activity that you like.

Physical activity can be especially helpful in bringing down insulin after a meal. Regular activity can also help improve your mood and boost your energy. If you aren't very active now, buildup slowly. Work toward moving for at least 60 minutes every day. Making physical activity fun is the key to keeping it an ongoing part of your life.

(Source: "Living Well With Polycystic Ovary Syndrome (PCOS)," girlshealth.gov, Office on Women's Health (OWH).)

What If I Have Worries About PCOS?

If you have been told you have PCOS, you may feel frustrated or sad. You may also feel relieved that at last there is an explanation for the problems you've been having. At the same time, having a diagnosis without an easy cure can be difficult.

Keep in mind that there are treatments for many of the problems that PCOS can cause. It is important to find a doctor who knows a lot about PCOS. You also want to feel comfortable with that person. Also, try to keep a positive attitude. And working on a healthy lifestyle, even when results take a long time, can help a lot, too!

Remember that you are not alone. Many girls with PCOS say that talking with a counselor about their concerns can be very helpful.

Having a healthy lifestyle through ups and downs is the first step to living well with PCOS!

Chapter 9

Psychological Effects Of Acne

What Is Acne?

Acne is a common skin disorder characterized by blackheads, whiteheads, nodules, or cysts on the face and upper body. Attributed to the clogging of oil glands in the skin, acne affects around 85 percent of young people between the ages of 12 and 25. Cases can range from mild (occasional outbreaks near the skin's surface that resolve easily) to severe (sustained outbreaks of nodules and cysts deep in the skin that can cause scarring). However, most acne can be treated effectively by medical professionals and the condition generally resolves itself as an individual moves away from adolescence and into adulthood.

Because acne occurs at a time in a person's life when they are establishing their own self-image and learning how to interact with others, the condition can negatively impact their emotional and psychological wellbeing. Periodic or sustained feelings of low self-esteem, anxiety, and depression are not uncommon in people with acne.

Psychological Impact Of Acne

For teens, having acne is an emotionally challenging experience. The condition often impacts their self-esteem, confidence, and mood, which in turn affects their school work, social life, and outlook on world around them. They tend to shy away from social events, interaction with their peers, and can become reclusive. In some severe cases, the emotional impact of acne can lead to depression. Symptoms of depression include feelings of worthlessness, excessive crying, withdrawal from family and friends, disturbances in sleeping or eating patterns, and

---

academic problems. If you or someone around you is experiencing these symptoms, you should seek out help from a parent or professional as early as possible.

It's also important to note that each person copes differently with emotional challenges of acne. The severity of the condition, a person's age and gender, what support systems they have, and where they are at in their overall emotional development can have an impact on their coping skills.

Social Impact Of Acne

During the teen years, individuals are learning how to interact with others and the world around them. Therefore, feelings of low self-esteem stemming from acne can have a significant impact on body image, sexuality, and social development. These impacts can include:

Social Withdrawal

- Teens with acne may not have the confidence to socialize with their peers or with others.

- Fear of rejection because of their appearance may keep some teens from interacting with members of the opposite sex or dating.

- Taunts from others about acne may induce individuals to withdraw completely from social interactions.

Education And Work

The low self-esteem experienced by individuals with acne can also affect their education and work. Teens with acne may skip school to keep from being seen, which in turn affects their grades. Employees may lack the self-confidence to excel in their work or take more sick days. Studies have also suggested that prospective employees who suffer from acne have a more difficult time finding a job since low self-esteem affects their job interviews.

Treatment And Management Of Acne

Lessening the psychological burden of acne is directly related to treating the condition itself. Many treatments exist today that effectively control acne and minimize any potential scarring. A medial professional can work with teens to create a program that works best for them and their particular case. It is also equally important not to dismiss the real emotional and psychological impact of acne. Parents and medical professionals can help teens overcome the stigma and negative thinking that can arise from the condition. They can also help identify signs of depression and make sure the teens suffering from depression gets the help they need as quickly as possible.

References

1. "Effect Of Acne Vulgaris On Quality Of Life Of Teenagers Compared To Parent Perceived Effect On Quality Of Life," ClinicalTrials.gov, National Institutes of Health (NIH), January 2016.

2. "Acne," National Women's Health Information Center (NWHIC), Office on Women's Health (OWH), July 16, 2009.

3. "Psychological Impairments In The Patients With Acne," National Center for Biotechnology Information (NCBI), January 2013.

4. "Knowledge, Beliefs, And Psychosocial Effect Of Acne Vulgaris Among Saudi Acne Patients," National Center for Biotechnology Information (NCBI), December 9, 2013.

5. "Acne: More Than Skin Deep," National Center for Biotechnology Information (NCBI), August 2006.

6. "The Psychosocial Impact Of Acne Vulgaris," National Center for Biotechnology Information (NCBI), September 2016.

7. "Psychological Effects Of Acne," DermNet New Zealand, February 2014.

8. "Acne," American Academy of Dermatology, n.d.

Part Three
Infectious Conditions Of The Skin

Chapter 10

Bacterial Infections: Cellulitis, Impetigo, Necrotizing Fasciitis, And Staphylococcal Infections

Bacterial Infections

Bacteria are living things that have only one cell. Under a microscope, they look like balls, rods, or spirals. They are so small that a line of 1,000 could fit across a pencil eraser. Most bacteria won't hurt you—less than 1 percent of the different types make people sick. Many are helpful. Some bacteria help to digest food, destroy disease-causing cells, and give the body needed vitamins. Bacteria are also used in making healthy foods like yogurt and cheese.

But infectious bacteria can make you ill. They reproduce quickly in your body. Many give off chemicals called toxins, which can damage tissue and make you sick. Examples of bacteria that cause infections include *Streptococcus, Staphylococcus, and E. coli.*

Antibiotics are the usual treatment. When you take antibiotics, follow the directions carefully. Each time you take antibiotics, you increase the chances that bacteria in your body will

About This Chapter: Text under the heading "Bacterial Infections" is excerpted from "Bacterial Infections," MedlinePlus, National Institutes of Health (NIH), August 25, 2014; Text under the heading "Cellulitis" is excerpted from "Cellulitis," MedlinePlus, National Institutes of Health (NIH), August 30, 2016; Text under the heading "Treatment" is excerpted from "Antimicrobial Stewardship Guidance," Bureau of Prisons (BOP), March 2013. Reviewed August 2017; Text under the heading "Impetigo" is excerpted from "How To Treat Impetigo And Control This Common Skin Infection," U.S. Food and Drug Administration (FDA), November 1, 2016; Text under the heading "Necrotizing Fasciitis" is excerpted from "Necrotizing Fasciitis: A Rare Disease, Especially For The Healthy," Centers for Disease Control and Prevention (CDC), July 3, 2017; Text under the heading "Staphylococcal Infections" is excerpted from "Staphylococcal Infections," MedlinePlus, National Institutes of Health (NIH), August 25, 2016; Text under the heading "Treatment" is excerpted from "Staph Infections," Centers for Disease Control and Prevention (CDC), October 28, 2009. Reviewed August 2017.

learn to resist them causing antibiotic resistance. Later, you could get or spread an infection that those antibiotics cannot cure.

Cellulitis

Cellulitis is an infection of the skin and deep underlying tissues. Group A strep (streptococcal) bacteria are the most common cause. The bacteria enter your body when you get an injury such as a bruise, burn, surgical cut, or wound.

Symptoms include:

- Fever and chills
- Swollen glands or lymph nodes
- A rash with painful, red, tender skin. The skin may blister and scab over.

Your healthcare provider may take a sample or culture from your skin or do a blood test to identify the bacteria causing infection. Treatment is with antibiotics. They may be oral in mild cases, or intravenous (by IV) for more severe cases.

Treatment

Mild:

- Penicillin
- Clindamycin

Moderate:

- SMX-TMP
- Clindamycin
- levofloxacin OR moxifloxacin

Severe:

- Vancomycin PLUS one of the following:
  - Ampicillin-sulbactam
  - Piperacillin-tazobactam
  - Ticarcillin-clavulanate
  - Metronidazole.)
  - Linezolid

Impetigo

It's a scary sight when your child comes home from daycare or elementary school with red sores and oozing fluid-filled blisters. Don't be alarmed if it's impetigo. Impetigo—one of the most common childhood diseases—can be treated with medications approved by the U.S. Food and Drug Administration (FDA).

Impetigo is a common bacterial skin infection that can produce blisters or sores anywhere on the body, but usually on the face (around the nose and mouth), neck, hands, and diaper area. It's contagious, preventable, and manageable with antibiotics, says pediatrician Thomas D. Smith, MD, of FDA.

What Causes Impetigo

Two types of bacteria found on our skin cause impetigo: *Staphylococcus aureus* and *Streptococcus pyogenes* (which also causes strep throat). Most of us go about our lives carrying around these bacteria without a problem, Smith says. But then a minor cut, scrape or insect bite allows the bacteria to cause an infection, resulting in impetigo.

Anyone can get impetigo—and more than once, Smith says. Although impetigo is a year-round disease, it occurs most often during the warm weather months. There are more than 3 million cases of impetigo in the United States every year.

"We typically see impetigo with kids 2 to 6 years old, probably because they get more cuts and scrapes and scratch more. And that spreads the bacteria," Smith says.

Treating Impetigo

Look for these signs of impetigo:

- itchy red sores that fill with fluid and then burst open, forming a yellow crust
- itchy rash
- fluid-filled blisters

If you see those symptoms, visit your healthcare provider. Impetigo is usually treated with topical or oral antibiotics. If you have multiple lesions or if there is an outbreak, your doctor might prescribe an oral antibiotic. There is no over-the-counter (OTC) treatment for impetigo.

Controlling And Preventing Impetigo

Untreated, impetigo often clears up on its own after a few days or weeks, Smith says. The key is to keep the infected area clean with soap and water and not to scratch it. The downside of not treating impetigo is that some people might develop more lesions that spread to other areas of their body.

And you can infect others. "To spread impetigo, you need fairly close contact—not casual contact—with the infected person or the objects they touched," he says. Avoid spreading impetigo to other people or other parts of your body by:

- Cleaning the infected areas with soap and water.
- Loosely covering scabs and sores until they heal.
- Gently removing crusty scabs.
- Washing your hands with soap and water after touching infected areas or infected persons.

Because impetigo spreads by skin-to-skin contact, there often are small outbreaks within a family or a classroom, Smith says. Avoid touching objects that someone with impetigo has used, such as utensils, towels, sheets, clothing and toys. If you have impetigo, keep your fingernails short so the bacteria can't live under your nails and spread. Also, don't scratch the sores.

Call your healthcare provider if the symptoms don't go away or if there are signs the infection has worsened, such as fever, pain, or increased swelling.

Necrotizing Fasciitis

Necrotizing fasciitis is a serious bacterial skin infection that spreads quickly and kills the body's soft tissue. (Necrotizing means "causing the death of tissues.") Accurate diagnosis, prompt treatment with antibiotics (medicines that kill bacteria in the body) through a vein, and surgery are important to stopping this infection that can become life-threatening in a very short amount of time.

Commonly called a "flesh-eating infection" by the media, this rare disease can be caused by more than one type of bacteria. These include group A *Streptococcus* (group A strep), *Klebsiella*, *Clostridium*, *Escherichia coli*, *Staphylococcus aureus*, and *Aeromonas hydrophila*, among others. Group A strep is considered the most common cause of necrotizing fasciitis.

Usually, infections from group A strep bacteria are generally mild and are easily treated. But in cases of necrotizing fasciitis, bacteria spread rapidly once they enter the body. They infect flat layers of a membrane known as the *fascia*, which are connective bands of tissue that surround muscles, nerves, fat, and blood vessels. The infection also damages the tissues next to the fascia. Sometimes toxins (poisons) made by these bacteria destroy the tissue they infect, causing it to die. When this happens, the infection is very serious and can result in loss of limbs or death.

> If you're healthy, have a strong immune system, and practice good hygiene and proper wound care, your chances of getting necrotizing fasciitis ("flesh-eating" bacteria) are extremely low.

Good Wound Care Is Important

What Are Wounds?

Wounds are injuries that break the skin or other body tissues. They include cuts, scrapes, scratches, and punctured skin. They often happen because of an accident, but surgery, sutures, and stitches also cause wounds. Minor wounds usually aren't serious, but it is important to clean them. Serious and infected wounds may require first aid followed by a visit to your doctor. You should also seek attention if the wound is deep, you cannot close it yourself, you cannot stop the bleeding or get the dirt out, or it does not heal.

(Source: "Wounds And Injuries," MedlinePlus, National Institutes of Health (NIH).)

Common sense and good wound care are the best ways to prevent a bacterial skin infection.

- Keep draining or open wounds covered with clean, dry bandages until healed.

- Don't delay first aid of even minor, noninfected wounds like blisters, scrapes, or any break in the skin.

- If you have an open wound or active infection, avoid spending time in whirlpools, hot tubs, swimming pools, and natural bodies of water (e.g., lakes, rivers, oceans) until infections are healed.

- Wash hands often with soap and water or use an alcohol-based hand rub if washing is not possible.

Necrotizing Fasciitis Is Rarely Spread From Person To Person

Most cases of necrotizing fasciitis occur randomly and are not linked to similar infections in others. The most common way of getting necrotizing fasciitis is when the bacteria enter the body through a break in the skin, like a cut, scrape, burn, insect bite, or puncture wound.

Most people who get necrotizing fasciitis have other health problems that may lower their body's ability to fight infection. Some of these conditions include diabetes, kidney disease, cancer, or other chronic health conditions that weaken the body's immune system. If you're healthy, have a strong immune system, and practice good hygiene and proper wound care, your chances of getting necrotizing fasciitis are extremely low.

Symptoms Can Often Be Confusing

The symptoms often start within hours after an injury and may seem like another illness or injury. Some people infected with necrotizing fasciitis may complain of pain or soreness, similar to that of a "pulled muscle." The skin may be warm with red or purplish areas of swelling that spread rapidly. There may be ulcers, blisters, or black spots on the skin. Patients often describe their pain as severe and way out of proportion to how the painful area looks when examined by a doctor. Fever, chills, fatigue (tiredness), or vomiting may follow the initial wound or soreness. These confusing symptoms may delay a person from seeking medical attention. If you think you may have these symptoms after a wound, see a doctor right away.

Prompt Treatment Is Needed

The first line of defense against this disease is strong antibiotics given through a needle into a vein. But because the bacterial toxins can destroy soft tissue and reduce blood flow, antibiotics may not reach all of the infected and dying areas. This is why rapid surgical exploration and removal of dead tissue—in addition to antibiotics—is often critical to stopping the infection.

Staphylococcal Infections

Staph is short for *Staphylococcus*, a type of bacteria. There are over 30 types, but *Staphylococcus aureus* causes most staph infections (pronounced "staff infections"), including:

- Skin infections

- Pneumonia

- Food poisoning

- Toxic shock syndrome

- Blood poisoning (bacteremia)

Skin infections are the most common. They can look like pimples or boils. They may be red, swollen and painful, and sometimes have pus or other drainage. They can turn into impetigo, which turns into a crust on the skin, or cellulitis, a swollen, red area of skin that feels hot.

Anyone can get a staph skin infection. You are more likely to get one if you have a cut or scratch, or have contact with a person or surface that has staph bacteria. The best way to prevent staph is to keep hands and wounds clean. Most staph skin infections are easily treated with antibiotics or by draining the infection. Some staph bacteria such as MRSA (methicillin-resistant *Staphylococcus aureus*) are resistant to certain antibiotics, making infections harder to treat.

Treatment

If you do get a staph infection, and get an antibiotic (medicine), it is important to take your antibiotic until it is finished, even if you are feeling better. If you don't, the staph germ may become resistant to the antibiotic.

How To Prevent Spreading Staphylococcal Infections?

- Cover your wounds. Keep wounds covered with clean, dry bandages until healed. Follow your doctor's instructions about proper care of the wound. Keeping the infection covered will help prevent the spread to others. Bandages and tape can be thrown away with the regular trash. Do not try to treat the infection yourself by picking or popping the sore.

- Clean your hands often. You, your family, and others in close contact should wash their hands often with soap and water or use an alcohol-based hand rub, especially after changing the bandage or touching the infected wound.

- Do not share personal items. Personal items include towels, washcloths, razors and clothing, including uniforms.

- Wash used sheets, towels, and clothes with water and laundry detergent. Use a dryer to dry them completely.

- Wash clothes according to manufacturer's instructions on the label. Clean your hands after touching dirty clothes.

(Source: "General Information About MRSA In The Community," Centers for Disease Control and Prevention (CDC).)

Chapter 11

Pseudomonas Dermatitis (Hot Tub Rash)

If contaminated water comes in contact with a person's skin for a long period of time, it can cause a rash called hot tub rash, or dermatitis. Hot tub rash is often caused by infection with the germ *Pseudomonas aeruginosa*. This germ is common in the environment (for example, in the water and soil) and is microscopic, so it can't be seen with the naked eye.

What Are The Symptoms Of Hot Tub Rash?

Symptoms of hot tub rash include:

- Itchy spots on the skin that become a bumpy red rash.
- The rash is worse in areas that were previously covered by a swimsuit.
- Pus-filled blisters around hair follicles.

Hot tub rash can affect people of all ages. Most rashes clear up in a few days without medical treatment. However, if your rash lasts longer than a few days, consult your healthcare provider.

How Is Hot Tub Rash Spread At Recreational Water Venues?

Hot tub rash can occur if contaminated water comes in contact with skin for a long period of time. The rash usually appears within a few days of being in a poorly maintained hot tub (or

---

About This Chapter: This chapter includes text excerpted from "Rashes" Centers for Disease Control and Prevention (CDC), May 4, 2016.

spa), but it can also appear within a few days after swimming in a poorly maintained pool or contaminated lake. Most rashes clear up in a few days without medical treatment. However, if your rash lasts longer than a few days, consult your healthcare provider.

How Do I Protect Myself And My Family?

Heed...Hot Tub Rules For Safe And Healthy Use

- Don't enter a hot tub when you have diarrhea.
- Don't swallow hot tub water or even get it into your mouth.
- Shower or bathe with soap before entering the hot tub.
- Observe limits, if posted, on the maximum allowable number of bathers.
- Don't let children less than 5 years of age use hot tubs.
- Don't drink alcohol before entering the hot tub or during hot tub use.
- If pregnant, consult a physician before hot tub use, particularly in the first trimester.

(Source: "Hot Tub/Spa User Information," Centers for Disease Control and Prevention (CDC).)

Because hot tubs have warmer water than pools, chlorine or other disinfectants used to kill germs (like Pseudomonas aeruginosa) break down faster. This can increase the risk of hot tub rash infection for swimmers.

To reduce the risk of hot tub rash:

- Remove your swimsuit and shower with soap after getting out of the water.

- Clean your swimsuit after getting out of the water.

- Ask your pool/hot tub operator if disinfectant (for example, chlorine) and pH levels are checked at least twice per day—hot tubs and pools with good disinfectant and pH control are less likely to spread germs.

- Use hot tub test strips to check the hot tub yourself for adequate disinfectant (chlorine or bromine) levels. CDC recommends the following for pools and hot tubs:

  - Pools: free chlorine (1–3 parts per million or ppm)

  - Hot Tubs: free chlorine (2–4 ppm) or bromine (4–6 ppm)

  - Both hot tubs and pools should have a pH level of 7.2–7.8

  - If you find improper chlorine, bromine, and/or pH levels, tell the hot tub/pool operator or owner immediately.

What Should You Notice?

- No odor; a well-chlorinated hot tub has little odor. A strong chemical smell indicates a maintenance problem.

- Smooth hot tub sides; tiles should not be sticky or slippery.

- Hot tub equipment is working; pumps and filtration systems make noise and you should hear them running.

- Hot tub temperature; the water temperature should not exceed 104°F (40°C)

- Check the hot tub water; test for adequate free chlorine (2–4 parts per million or ppm) or bromine (4–6 ppm) and pH (7.2–7.8) levels using hot tub test strips.

(Source: "Hot Tub/Spa User Information," Centers for Disease Control and Prevention (CDC).)

What Can I Ask The Hot Tub Operator?

- What was the most recent health inspection score for the hot tub?

- Are disinfectant and pH levels checked at least twice per day?

- Are disinfectant and pH levels checked more often when the hot tub is being used by a lot of people?

- Are the following maintenance activities performed regularly?

  - Removal of the slime or biofilm layer by scrubbing and cleaning?

  - Replacement of the hot tub water filter according to manufacturer's recommendations?

  - Replacement of hot tub water?

Chapter 12

Lyme Disease

While everyone is susceptible to tick bites, campers, hikers, and people who work on gardens and in other leafy outdoor venues are at the greatest risk of being bitten by them.

This is important because Lyme disease, an infection caused by the bacterium *Borrelia burgdorferi*, or *B. burgdorferi*, is transmitted via the bite of infected ticks.

Lyme disease is named after a town in Connecticut where, in 1975, it was first recognized. It is transmitted by a group of closely related species of ticks known as Ixodes.

Ticks in this group—deer ticks, western black-legged ticks, and black-legged ticks—are much smaller than the common dog or cattle ticks, and attach to any part of the body, often to moist or hairy areas such as the groin, armpits, and scalp.

The overwhelming majority of cases are reported in the summer months when ticks are most active and people spend more time outdoors.

The U.S. Food and Drug Administration (FDA) regulates products that are used to help diagnose and treat this complex disease in humans. There are no licensed vaccines in the United States to aid in the prevention of Lyme disease in people.

Here's a look at what you need to know to protect yourself.

What Are The Symptoms?

Lyme disease can cause fever, headaches, fatigue, and a characteristic skin rash called erythema migrans. Left untreated, infection can spread to joints, the heart, and the nervous

About This Chapter: This chapter includes text excerpted from "Beware Of Ticks ... & Lyme Disease," U.S. Food and Drug Administration (FDA), November 18, 2015.

system. Permanent damage to the joints or the nervous system can develop in patients with late Lyme disease. It is rarely, if ever, fatal.

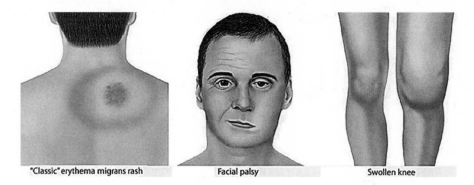

"Classic" erythema migrans rash   Facial palsy   Swollen knee

Figure 12.1. Areas Where Lyme Disease Occurs

(Source: "Signs And Symptoms Of Untreated Lyme Disease," Centers for Disease Control and Prevention (CDC).)

Lyme Disease Has Different Stages

Erythema migrans is a key early-stage symptom. This circular red patch usually appears at the bite site 3 to 30 days after the bite. It expands to 5 to 6 inches in diameter, and persists for 3 to 5 weeks. As the rash enlarges, it may take on a "bull's-eye" appearance. In some people this rash never forms, or it is not noticed.

Other symptoms of early Lyme disease include:

• muscle and joint aches

• headache

• chills and fever

• fatigue

• swollen lymph nodes

Other symptoms may not appear until weeks or months after a tick bite occurs. They include:

• arthritis (usually as pain and swelling in large joints, especially the knee)

• nervous system abnormalities

• heart-rhythm irregularities

What Precautions Can I Take?

Educate yourself about Lyme disease, and try not to get bitten by ticks. More specifically:

- Avoid wooded, brushy, and grassy areas, especially in May, June, and July. (Contact the local health department or park/extension service for information on the prevalence of ticks in specific areas.)

- Wear light-colored clothing so that you can see ticks that get on you.

- Wear long pants and long-sleeved shirts.

- Wear shoes that cover the entire foot.

- Tuck pant legs into socks or shoes, and tuck shirts into pants.

- Wear a hat for extra protection.

- Spray insect repellent containing N,N-Diethyl-*meta*-toluamide or DEET on clothes and exposed skin other than the face, or treat clothes with permethrin, which kills ticks on contact.

- Walk in the center of trails to avoid brush and grass.

- Remove your clothing, and wash and dry them at high temperatures after being outdoors.

- Do a careful body check for ticks after outdoor activities.

There's A Tick Attached To Me. What Do I Do?

Remove it! Using tweezers, grasp the tick close to the skin, pull straight back, and avoid crushing the tick's body. Save the tick for possible identification by a doctor or the local health department.

Steps For Removing A Tick
- Use fine-tipped tweezers to grasp the tick as close to the skin's surface as possible.
- Pull upward with steady, even pressure. Don't twist or jerk the tick; this can cause the mouth-parts to break off and remain in the skin. If this happens, remove the mouth-parts with tweezers. If you are unable to remove the mouth easily with clean tweezers, leave it alone and let the skin heal.

> - After removing the tick, thoroughly clean the bite area and your hands with rubbing alcohol, an iodine scrub, or soap and water.
> - Dispose of a live tick by submerging it in alcohol, placing it in a sealed bag/container, wrapping it tightly in tape, or flushing it down the toilet. Never crush a tick with your fingers.
>
> *(Source: "Tick Removal," Centers for Disease Control and Prevention (CDC).)*

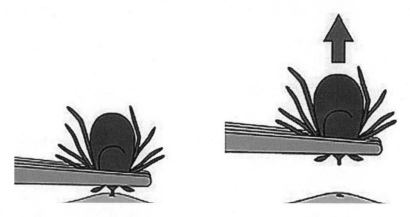

Figure 12.2. How To Remove A Tick

(Source: "Tick Removal," Centers for Disease Control and Prevention (CDC).)

I Think I May Have Lyme Disease. Now What?

There's diagnosis. And then there's treatment.

Diagnosis

Sally Hojvat, Ph.D., director of the Division of Microbiology Devices (DMD) at FDA's Center for Devices and Radiological Health (CDRH), says that health professionals need to consider the following while making a diagnosis of Lyme disease:

- a history of exposure to potentially infected ticks, especially in areas of the country known to have Lyme disease

- symptoms, including physical findings such as the characteristic rash

- results of blood tests that check for antibodies to the bacterium that causes Lyme disease.

About Blood Tests

- FDA regulates diagnostic tests for Lyme disease.

- Tests that use a blood sample for detecting antibodies to the bacterium that causes the disease have been cleared by FDA for commercial sale and distribution.

- Tests for Lyme disease that use urine or other body fluids to diagnose infection by the bacterium have not been cleared by FDA.

"It's important to know that blood tests that check for antibodies to the bacterium that causes Lyme disease are not useful if done soon after a tick bite," says Hojvat. "It takes 2 to 5 weeks after a tick bite for initial antibodies to develop."

There are two types of blood tests that should be performed on patients suspected of having Lyme disease, she says.

"The first is an ELISA (enzyme-linked immunosorbent assay) to measure antibody levels," Hojvat says. "The second test, the Western blot assay, identifies antibodies particular to the bacterium *B. burgdorferi*."

This approach is consistent with Centers for Disease Control and Prevention's (CDC's) recommended guidelines.

Treatment

According to CDC, patients treated with antibiotics in the early stages of the infection usually recover rapidly and completely.

Antibiotics commonly used for oral treatment include doxycycline, amoxicillin, or cefuroxime axetil (Ceftin). Patients with certain neurological or cardiac forms of illness may require intravenous treatment with drugs such as ceftriaxone or penicillin.

The National Institutes of Health (NIH) funded studies of longer courses of antibiotics for patients with some chronic symptoms several months after successful antibiotic therapy. Longer courses of antibiotic treatment have not been shown to be beneficial and have in fact been linked to serious complications, including death.

What About Pets?

Household pets can get Lyme disease, too. Typical symptoms in animals include joint soreness and lameness, fever, and loss of appetite.

Regularly checking pets for all types of ticks reduces the risk of infection for both pet and owner.

Preventing tick exposure with topical and/or collar products is very important in preventing Lyme disease in dogs.

Experts in FDA's Center for Veterinary Medicine (CVM) say that dogs with Lyme disease occasionally develop serious kidney disease that can be fatal.

CVM says there are two basic types of Lyme disease vaccines available for dogs: the killed bacteria and a genetically engineered (recombinant) vaccine. Talk to your veterinarian, since vaccinating against Lyme disease may not be appropriate for all dogs. There is no vaccine for cats, which do not seem to be susceptible to Lyme disease.

Chapter 13

Cold Sores And Canker Sores

What Are Cold Sores?

Cold sores are caused by a contagious virus called herpes simplex virus (HSV). There are two types of HSV. Type 1 usually causes oral herpes, or cold sores. Type 1 herpes virus infects more than half of the U.S. population by the time they reach their 20s. Type 2 usually affects the genital area

Some people have no symptoms from the infection. But others develop painful and unsightly cold sores. Cold sores usually occur outside the mouth, on or around the lips. When they are inside the mouth, they are usually on the gums or the roof of the mouth. They are not the same as canker sores, which are not contagious.

There is no cure for cold sores. They normally go away on their own in a few weeks. Antiviral medicines can help them heal faster. They can also help to prevent cold sores in people who often get them. Other medicines can help with the pain and discomfort of the sores. These include ointments that numb the blisters, soften the crusts of the sores, or dry them out. Protecting your lips from the sun with sunblock lip balm can also help.

What Are Canker Sores?

Canker sores are small, round sores in your mouth. They can be on the inside of your cheek, under your tongue, or in the back of your throat. They usually have a red edge and a gray center.

About This Chapter: Text under the heading "What Are Cold Sores?" is excerpted from "Cold Sores," MedlinePlus, National Institutes of Health (NIH), April 18, 2016; Text under the heading "What Are Canker Sores?" is excerpted from "Canker Sores," U.S. National Library of Medicine (NLM), National Institutes of Health (NIH), August 30, 2016.

They can be quite painful. They are not the same as cold sores, which are caused by herpes simplex.

Canker sores aren't contagious. They may happen if you have a viral infection. They may also be triggered by stress, food allergies, lack of vitamins and minerals, hormonal changes or menstrual periods. In some cases, the cause is unknown.

In most cases, the sores go away by themselves. Some ointments, creams or rinses may help with the pain. Avoiding hot, spicy food while you have a canker sore also helps.

Fever Blisters And Canker Sores

Fever blisters and canker sores are two of the most common disorders of the mouth, causing discomfort and annoyance to millions of Americans. Both cause small sores to develop in or around the mouth, and often are confused with each other. Canker sores, however, occur only inside the mouth—on the tongue and the inside linings of the cheeks, lips and throat. Fever blisters, also called cold sores, usually occur outside the mouth—on the lips, chin, cheeks or in the nostrils. When fever blisters do occur inside the mouth, it is usually on the gums or the roof of the mouth. Inside the mouth, fever blisters are smaller than canker sores, heal more quickly, and often begin as a blister.

(Source: "Fever Blisters And Canker Sores," National Institute of Dental and Craniofacial Research (NIDCR).)

Sutton Disease 2

Sutton disease 2, also known as recurrent aphthous stomatitis, is a chronic inflammatory disease characterized by painful ulcers in the mouth. These sores, which can be of varying size and frequency, are commonly called canker sores. The exact cause of this condition is not fully understood, although it may be due to an abnormal immune response. Treatment is not always necessary, but may include mouth rinses, topical ointments or systemic corticosteroids.

(Source: "Sutton Disease 2," Genetic and Rare Diseases Information Center (GARD), National Center for Advancing Translational Sciences (NCATS).)

Chapter 14

Human Papillomavirus (HPV) And Genital Warts

Human Papillomavirus (HPV)

What Is HPV?

HPV is short for human papillomavirus. HPV is a group of more than 150 related viruses. Each HPV virus in this large group is given a number which is called its HPV type. HPV is named for the warts (papillomas) some HPV types can cause. Some other HPV types can lead to cancer. Men and women can get cancer of mouth/ throat, and anus/rectum caused by HPV infections. Men can also get penile HPV cancer. In women, HPV infection can also cause cervical, vaginal, and vulvar HPV cancers. But there are vaccines that can prevent infection with the types of HPV that most commonly cause cancer.

How Do People Get HPV?

HPV is transmitted through intimate skin-to-skin contact. You can get HPV by having vaginal, anal, or oral sex with someone who has the virus. It is most commonly spread during vaginal or anal sex. HPV is so common that nearly all men and women get it at some point in their lives. HPV can be passed even when an infected person has no signs or symptoms. You can develop symptoms years after being infected, making it hard to know when you first became infected.

About This Chapter: Text under the heading "Human Papillomavirus (HPV)" is excerpted from "Human Papillomavirus (HPV)," Centers for Disease Control and Prevention (CDC), November 21, 2016; Text under the heading "Genital Warts" is excerpted from "Genital Warts," Office on Women's Health (OWH), U.S. Department of Health and Human Services (HHS), June 12, 2017.

In most cases, HPV goes away on its own and does not cause any health problems. But when HPV does not go away, it can cause health problems like genital warts and cancer.

Genital warts usually appear as a small bump or groups of bumps in the genital area. They can be small or large, raised or flat, or shaped like a cauliflower. A healthcare provider can usually diagnose warts by looking at the genital area.

HPV cancers include cancer of the cervix, vulva, vagina, penis, or anus. HPV infection can also cause cancer in the back of the throat, including the base of the tongue and tonsils.

How Common Are HPV Infections?

HPV infections are so common that nearly all men and women will get at least one type of HPV at some point in their lives. Most people never know that they have been infected and may give HPV to a sex partner without knowing it. About 79 million Americans are currently infected with some type of HPV. About 14 million people in the United States become newly infected each year.

What Kinds Of Problems Does HPV Infection Cause?

Most people with HPV never develop symptoms or health problems. Most HPV infections (9 out of 10) go away by themselves within two years. But, sometimes, HPV infections will last longer, and can cause certain cancers and other diseases. HPV infections can cause:

- cancers of the cervix, vagina, and vulva in women;

- cancers of the penis in men; and

- cancers of the anus and back of the throat, including the base of the tongue and tonsils (oropharynx), in both women and men. Every year in the United States, HPV causes 30,700 cancers in men and women.

How Do People Get An HPV Infection?

People get HPV from another person during intimate sexual contact. Most of the time, people get HPV from having vaginal and/or anal sex. Men and women can also get HPV from having oral sex or other sex play. A person can get HPV even if their partner doesn't have any signs or symptoms of HPV infection. A person can have HPV even if years have passed since he or she had sexual contact with an infected person. Most people do not realize they are infected. They also don't know that they may be passing HPV to their sex partner(s). It is possible for someone to get more than one type of HPV.

It's not very common, but sometimes a pregnant woman with HPV can pass it to her baby during delivery. The child might develop recurrent respiratory papillomatosis (RRP), a rare but dangerous condition where warts caused by HPV (similar to genital warts) grow inside the throat.

There haven't been any documented cases of people getting HPV from surfaces in the environment, such as toilet seats. However, someone could be exposed to HPV from objects (toys) shared during sexual activity if the object has been used by an infected person.

Who Should Get HPV Vaccine?

All girls and boys who are 11 or 12 years old should get the recommended series of HPV vaccine. The vaccination series can be started at age 9 years. Teen boys and girls who did not get vaccinated when they were younger should get it now. HPV vaccine is recommended for young women through age 26, and young men through age 21. HPV vaccine is also recommended for the following people, if they did not get vaccinated when they were younger:

- young men who have sex with men, including young men who identify as gay or bisexual or who intend to have sex with men through age 26;

- young adults who are transgender through age 26; and

- young adults with certain immunocompromising conditions (including HIV) through age 26.

> The HPV vaccine is licensed, safe, and effective for females and males ages 9 through 26, and the Advisory Committee on Immunization Practices (ACIP) recommends that all adolescents (males and females) begin receiving the vaccine at age 11 or 12. The Centers for Disease Control and Prevention's (CDC) Vaccines for Children Program (VFC) provides vaccines at no cost to over 40 million children under 19 each year.
>
> *(Source: "Adolescent Development & STDs," Office of Adolescent Health (OAH), U.S. Department of Health and Human Services (HHS).)*

Why Are Two Doses Recommended For 9–14 Year Olds, While Older Adolescents Need Three Doses?

HPV vaccines are recommended in a three-dose series given over six months. In 2016, Centers for Disease Control and Prevention (CDC) changed the recommendation to two doses for persons starting the series before their 15th birthday. The second dose of HPV vaccine should be given six to twelve months after the first dose. Adolescents who receive their two doses less than five months apart will require a third dose of HPV vaccine.

Teens and young adults who start the series at ages 15 through 26 years still need three doses of HPV vaccine Also, three doses are still recommended for people with certain immunocompromising conditions aged 9 through 26 years.

Studies have shown that two doses of HPV vaccine given at least six months apart to adolescents at age 9–14 years worked as well or better than three doses given to older adolescents and young adults.

Why Is HPV Vaccine Recommended At Age 11 Or 12 Years?

For HPV vaccine to be most effective, the series should be given prior to exposure to HPV. There is no reason to wait to vaccinate until teens reach puberty or start having sex. Preteens should receive all recommended doses of the HPV vaccine series long before they begin any type of sexual activity.

What Are The Possible Side Effects Of HPV Vaccination?

Vaccines, like any medicine, can have side effects. Many people who get HPV vaccine have no side effects at all. Some people report having very mild side effects, like a sore arm. The most common side effects are usually mild. Common side effects of HPV vaccine include:

- Pain, redness, or swelling in the arm where the shot was given
- Fever
- Headache or feeling tired
- Nausea
- Muscle or joint pain

Not getting HPV vaccine leaves people vulnerable to HPV infection and related cancers. Treatments for cancers and precancers might include surgery, chemotherapy, and/or radiation, which might cause pregnancy complications or leave someone unable to have children.

Genital Warts

What Are Genital Warts?

Genital warts are a type of sexually transmitted infection (STI) caused by the human papillomavirus (HPV). While there is no cure for HPV, you can get treated for genital warts.

Genital warts appear as a small bump or group of bumps in the genital area. Some genital warts are so small you cannot see them.

Who Gets Genital Warts?

About 400,000 Americans get genital warts each year. Researchers estimate that genital warts are more common in men.

How Do You Get Genital Warts?

Nearly all cases of genital warts are caused by HPV.

Genital warts are spread most often through direct skin-to-skin contact during vaginal or anal sex. HPV, the virus that causes genital warts, can be spread even if the person does not have any genital warts that you can see.

Rarely, genital warts are spread:

- By giving oral sex to someone who has HPV or genital warts

- By receiving oral sex from someone who has HPV or genital warts on his or her mouth, lips, or tongue

- During childbirth from a woman to her baby

What Are The Signs And Symptoms Of Genital Warts?

Genital warts usually appear as a small bump or group of bumps in the genital area. They are flesh-colored and can be flat or look bumpy like cauliflower. Some genital warts are so small you cannot see them.

In women, genital warts can grow:

- Inside the vagina

- On the vulva, cervix, or groin

- In or around the anus

- On the lips, mouth, tongue, or throat (this is very rare)

In men, genital warts can grow:

- On the penis

- On the scrotum, thigh, or groin

- In or around the anus

- On the lips, mouth, tongue, or throat (this is very rare)

Genital warts can cause itching, burning, and discomfort. Talk to your doctor if you think you have genital warts.

How Long Does It Take For Genital Warts To Appear?

Warts usually appear within months after having sexual contact with someone with the HPV types that cause genital warts. Sometimes the warts appear in just days or weeks, while other people do not show genital warts until years later. Some people may get HPV but never get genital warts.

How Are Genital Warts Treated?

There is no cure for HPV, but genital warts can be removed. If you decide to have warts removed, do not use over-the-counter medicines meant for other kinds of warts. There are special, prescription-only treatments for genital warts. Your doctor or nurse must prescribe the medicine for you.

Your doctor or nurse may apply a chemical to treat the warts in the doctor's office, or prescribe a cream for you to apply at home. Surgery is also an option. Your doctor may:

- Use an electric current to burn off the warts

- Use a light/laser to destroy warts

- Freeze off the warts

- Cut out the warts

Treatment can only remove the genital wart. Treatment does not cure HPV, the virus that causes genital warts.

Do I Have To Treat Genital Warts?

No. Some people choose not to treat genital warts. If left untreated, genital warts may go away, stay the same, or grow in size and number. Genital warts will not turn into cancer.

Even if you treat the genital warts, you can still spread genital warts and HPV, the virus that causes genital warts, to other people. Doctors do not know how long you are contagious after warts appear.

Could I Still Have Human Papillomavirus (HPV) If I Get My Genital Warts Removed?

Yes. Even when warts are treated, you may still have HPV. This is why warts can come back after treatment. You can still spread HPV to other people after genital warts are removed.

How Can I Prevent Genital Warts?

The best way to prevent genital warts or any STI is to not have vaginal, oral, or anal sex.

If you do have sex, lower your risk of getting an STI with the following steps:

- Get vaccinated

- Use condoms

- Get tested

- Be monogamous

- Limit your number of sex partners

- Do not douche

- Do not abuse alcohol or drugs

The steps work best when used together. No single step can protect you from every single type of STI.

Chapter 15

Varicella (Chickenpox And Shingles)

What Is Chickenpox?

Chickenpox is a very contagious disease caused by the varicella-zoster virus (VZV). It causes a blister-like rash, itching, tiredness, and fever. The rash appears first on the stomach, back and face and can spread over the entire body causing between 250 and 500 itchy blisters. Chickenpox can be serious, especially in babies, adults, and people with weakened immune systems. The best way to prevent chickenpox is to get the chickenpox vaccine.

Signs And Symptoms

Anyone who hasn't had chickenpox or gotten the chickenpox vaccine can get the disease. Chickenpox illness usually lasts about 5 to 7 days.

The classic symptom of chickenpox is a rash that turns into itchy, fluid-filled blisters that eventually turn into scabs. The rash may first show up on the face, chest, and back then spread to the rest of the body, including inside the mouth, eyelids, or genital area. It usually takes about one week for all the blisters to become scabs.

Other typical symptoms that may begin to appear 1–2 days before rash include:

- fever

- tiredness

About This Chapter: Text under the heading "What Is Chickenpox?" is excerpted from "Chickenpox (Varicella)," Centers for Disease Control and Prevention (CDC), July 1, 2016; Text under the heading "What Is Shingles?" is excerpted from "Shingles (Herpes Zoster)," Centers for Disease Control and Prevention (CDC), August 19, 2016.

- loss of appetite

- headache

Children usually miss 5 to 6 days of school or child care due to chickenpox.

Vaccinated Persons

Some people who have been vaccinated against chickenpox can still get the disease. However, the symptoms are usually milder with fewer red spots or blisters and mild or no fever. Though uncommon, some vaccinated people who get chickenpox will develop illness as serious as chickenpox in unvaccinated persons.

People at Risk for Severe Chickenpox

Some people who get chickenpox may have more severe symptoms and may be at higher risk for complications.

Complications

Complications from chickenpox can occur, but they are not common in healthy people who get the disease.

People who may get a serious case of chickenpox and may be at high risk for complications include:

- Infants

- Adolescents

- Adults

- Pregnant women

- People with weakened immune systems because of illness or medications; for example,

  - People with human immunodeficiency virus (HIV)/acquired immune deficiency syndrome (AIDS) or cancer.

  - Patients who have had transplants, and

  - People on chemotherapy, immunosuppressive medications, or long-term use of steroids.

Serious complications from chickenpox include:

- bacterial infections of the skin and soft tissues in children including Group A streptococcal infections

- pneumonia

- infection or inflammation of the brain (encephalitis, cerebellar ataxia)

- bleeding problems

- blood stream infections (sepsis)

- dehydration

Some people with serious complications from chickenpox can become so sick that they need to be hospitalized. Chickenpox can also cause death.

Some deaths from chickenpox continue to occur in healthy, unvaccinated children and adults. Many of the healthy adults who died from chickenpox contracted the disease from their unvaccinated children.

Transmission

Chickenpox is a very contagious disease caused by the varicella-zoster virus. The virus spreads easily from people with chickenpox to others who have never had the disease or been vaccinated. The virus spreads mainly by touching or breathing in the virus particles that come from chickenpox blisters, and possibly through tiny droplets from infected people that get into the air after they breathe or talk, for example.

The varicella-zoster virus also causes shingles. Chickenpox can be spread from people with shingles to others who have never had chickenpox or received the chickenpox vaccine. This can happen if a person touches or breathes in virus from shingles blisters. In these cases, a person might develop chickenpox, not shingles.

When Is A Person Contagious?

A person with chickenpox can spread the disease from 1 to 2 days before they get the rash until all their chickenpox blisters have formed scabs (usually 5–7 days).

It takes about 2 weeks (from 10 to 21 days) after exposure to a person with chickenpox or shingles for someone to develop chickenpox.

If a person vaccinated for chickenpox gets the disease, they can still spread it to others.

For most people, getting chickenpox once provides immunity for life. However, for a few people, they can get chickenpox more than once, although this is not common.

Prevention

The best way to prevent chickenpox is to get the chickenpox vaccine. Children, adolescents, and adults should get two doses of chickenpox vaccine.

Chickenpox vaccine is very safe and effective at preventing the disease. Most people who get the vaccine will not get chickenpox. If a vaccinated person does get chickenpox, it is usually mild—with fewer red spots or blisters and mild or no fever. The chickenpox vaccine prevents almost all cases of severe disease.

Two doses of the vaccine are about 90 percent effective at preventing chickenpox. When you get vaccinated, you protect yourself and others in your community. This is especially important for people who cannot get vaccinated, such as those with weakened immune systems or pregnant women.

For people exposed to chickenpox, call a healthcare provider if the person:

- has never had chickenpox disease and is not vaccinated with the chickenpox vaccine

- is pregnant

- has a weakened immune system caused by disease or medication; for example,

  - People with HIV/AIDS or cancer

  - Patients who have had transplants, and

  - People on chemotherapy, immunosuppressive medications, or long-term use of steroids

Treatments

There are several things that can be done at home to help relieve the symptoms and prevent skin infections. Calamine lotion and colloidal oatmeal baths may help relieve some of the itching. Keeping fingernails trimmed short may help prevent skin infections caused by scratching blisters.

Over-The-Counter Medications

Use nonaspirin medications, such as acetaminophen, to relieve fever from chickenpox.

Do not use aspirin or aspirin-containing products to relieve fever from chickenpox. The use of aspirin in children with chickenpox has been associated with Reye syndrome, a severe disease that affects the liver and brain and can cause death.

When To Call The Healthcare Provider

Some people are more likely to have a serious case of chickenpox. Call a healthcare provider if:

1. the person at risk of serious complications:

    *   is less than 1 year-old

    *   is older than 12 years of age

    *   has a weakened immune system

    *   is pregnant, or

2. develops any of the following symptoms:

    *   fever that lasts longer than 4 days

    *   fever that rises above 102°F (38.9°C)

    *   any areas of the rash or any part of the body becomes very red, warm, or tender, or begins leaking pus (thick, discolored fluid), since these symptoms may indicate a bacterial infection

    *   extreme illness

    *   difficult waking up or confused demeanor

    *   difficulty walking

    *   stiff neck

    *   frequent vomiting

    *   difficulty breathing

    *   severe cough

    *   severe abdominal pain

    *   rash with bleeding or bruising (hemorrhagic rash)

Treatments Prescribed By Your Doctor For People With Chickenpox

Your healthcare provider can advise you on treatment options. Antiviral medications are recommended for people with chickenpox who are more likely to develop serious disease including:

*   otherwise healthy people older than 12 years of age

- people with chronic skin or lung disease

- people receiving steroid therapy

- pregnant women

Acyclovir, an antiviral medication, is licensed for treatment of chickenpox. The medication works best if it is given within the first 24 hours after the rash starts.

What Is Shingles?

Almost 1 out of every 3 people in the United States will develop shingles, also known as zoster or herpes zoster, in their lifetime. There are an estimated 1 million cases of shingles each year in this country. Anyone who has recovered from chickenpox may develop shingles; even children can get shingles. However the risk of shingles increases as you get older. About half of all cases occur in men and women 60 years old or older.

Some people have a greater risk of getting shingles. This includes people who:

- have medical conditions that keep their immune systems from working properly, such as certain cancers like leukemia and lymphoma, and human immunodeficiency virus (HIV), and

- receive immunosuppressive drugs, such as steroids and drugs that are given after organ transplantation.

People who develop shingles typically have only one episode in their lifetime. However, a person can have a second or even a third episode.

Cause

Shingles is caused by the varicella zoster virus (VZV), the same virus that causes chickenpox. After a person recovers from chickenpox, the virus stays dormant (inactive) in the body. For reasons that are not fully known, the virus can reactivate years later, causing shingles. Shingles is not caused by the same virus that causes genital herpes, a sexually transmitted disease.

Signs And Symptoms

Shingles is a painful rash that develops on one side of the face or body. The rash forms blisters that typically scab over in 7 to 10 days and clears up within 2 to 4 weeks.

Before the rash develops, people often have pain, itching, or tingling in the area where the rash will develop. This may happen anywhere from 1 to 5 days before the rash appears.

Most commonly, the rash occurs in a single stripe around either the left or the right side of the body. In other cases, the rash occurs on one side of the face. In rare cases (usually among people with weakened immune systems), the rash may be more widespread and look similar to a chickenpox rash. Shingles can affect the eye and cause loss of vision.

Other symptoms of shingles can include:

- Fever

- Headache

- Chills

- Upset stomach

Transmission

Shingles cannot be passed from one person to another. However, the virus that causes shingles, the varicella zoster virus, can be spread from a person with active shingles to another person who has never had chickenpox. In such cases, the person exposed to the virus might develop chickenpox, but they would not develop shingles

The virus is spread through direct contact with fluid from the rash blisters caused by shingles.

A person with active shingles can spread the virus when the rash is in the blister-phase. A person is not infectious before the blisters appear. Once the rash has developed crusts, the person is no longer contagious.

Shingles is less contagious than chickenpox and the risk of a person with shingles spreading the virus is low if the rash is covered.

If you have shingles:

- Keep the rash covered.

- Avoid touching or scratching the rash.

- Wash your hands often to prevent the spread of varicella zoster virus.

- Until your rash has developed crusts, avoid contact with:

  - pregnant women who have never had chickenpox or the chickenpox vaccine;

  - premature or low birth weight infants; and

  - people with weakened immune systems, such as people receiving immunosuppressive medications or undergoing chemotherapy, organ transplant recipients, and people with human immunodeficiency virus (HIV) infection.

Complications

The most common complication of shingles is a condition called postherpetic neuralgia (PHN). People with PHN have severe pain in the areas where they had the shingles rash, even after the rash clears up.

The pain from PHN may be severe and debilitating, but it usually resolves in a few weeks or months in most patients. Some people can have pain from PHN for many years.

As people get older, they are more likely to develop PHN, and the pain is more likely to be severe. PHN occurs rarely among people under 40 years of age but can occur in up to a third of untreated people who are 60 years of age and older.

Shingles may lead to serious complications involving the eye. Very rarely, shingles can also lead to pneumonia, hearing problems, blindness, brain inflammation (encephalitis), or death.

Prevention

The only way to reduce the risk of developing shingles and the long-term pain from postherpetic neuralgia (PHN) is to get vaccinated. Centers for Disease Control and Prevention (CDC) recommends that people aged 60 years and older get one dose of shingles vaccine. Shingles vaccine is available in pharmacies and doctor's offices. Talk with your healthcare professional if you have questions about shingles vaccine.

Treatment

Several antiviral medicines—acyclovir, valacyclovir, and famciclovir—are available to treat shingles. These medicines will help shorten the length and severity of the illness. But to be effective, they must be started as soon as possible after the rash appears. People who have or think they might have shingles should call their healthcare provider as soon as possible to discuss treatment options.

Analgesics (pain medicine) may help relieve the pain caused by shingles. Wet compresses, calamine lotion, and colloidal oatmeal baths may help relieve some of the itching.

Chapter 16

Molluscum Contagiosum

Molluscum contagiosum is an infection caused by a poxvirus (molluscum contagiosum virus). The result of the infection is usually a benign, mild skin disease characterized by lesions (growths) that may appear anywhere on the body. Within 6–12 months, Molluscum contagiosum typically resolves without scarring but may take as long as 4 years. The lesions, known as Mollusca, are small, raised, and usually white, pink, or flesh-colored with a dimple or pit in the center. They often have a pearly appearance. They're usually smooth and firm. In most people, the lesions range from about the size of a pinhead to as large as a pencil eraser (2 to 5 millimeters in diameter). They may become itchy, sore, red, and/or swollen. Mollusca may occur anywhere on the body including the face, neck, arms, legs, abdomen, and genital area, alone or in groups. The lesions are rarely found on the palms of the hands or the soles of the feet.

Transmission

The virus that causes molluscum spreads from direct person-to-person physical contact and through contaminated fomites. Fomites are inanimate objects that can become contaminated with virus; in the instance of molluscum contagiosum this can include linens such as clothing and towels, bathing sponges, pool equipment, and toys. Although the virus might be spread by sharing swimming pools, baths, saunas, or other wet and warm environments, this has not been proven. Researchers who have investigated this idea think it is more likely the virus is spread by sharing towels and other items around a pool or sauna than through water.

About This Chapter: This chapter includes text excerpted from "Molluscum Contagiosum," Centers for Disease Control and Prevention (CDC), May 11, 2015.

Someone with molluscum can spread it to other parts of their body by touching or scratching a lesion and then touching their body somewhere else. This is called autoinoculation. Shaving and electrolysis can also spread mollusca to other parts of the body.

Molluscum can spread from one person to another by sexual contact. Many, but not all, cases of molluscum in adults are caused by sexual contact.

Conflicting reports make it unclear whether the disease may be spread by simple contact with seemingly intact lesions or if the breaking of a lesion and the subsequent transferring of core material is necessary to spread the virus.

The molluscum contagiosum virus remains in the top layer of skin (epidermis) and does not circulate throughout the body; therefore, it cannot spread through coughing or sneezing. Since the virus lives only in the top layer of skin, once the lesions are gone the virus is gone and you cannot spread it to others. Molluscum contagiosum is not like herpes viruses, which can remain dormant ("sleeping") in your body for long periods and then reappear.

Risk Factors

Molluscum contagiosum is common enough that you should not be surprised if you see someone with it or if someone in your family becomes infected. Although not limited to children, it is most common in children 1 to 10 years of age. People at increased risk for getting the disease include:

- People with weakened immune systems (i.e., Human immunodeficiency virus (HIV) infected persons or persons being treated for cancer) are at higher risk for getting molluscum contagiosum. Their growths may look different, be larger, and be more difficult to treat.

- Atopic dermatitis may also be a risk factor for getting molluscum contagiosum due to frequent breaks in the skin. People with this condition also may be more likely to spread molluscum contagiousm to other parts of their body for the same reason.

- People who live in warm, humid climates where living conditions are crowded.

In addition, there is evidence that molluscum infections have been on the rise in the United States since 1966, but these infections are not routinely monitored because they are seldom serious and routinely disappear without treatment.

Treatment Options

Because molluscum contagiosum is self-limited in healthy individuals, treatment may be unnecessary. Nonetheless, issues such as lesion visibility, underlying atopic disease, and the desire to prevent transmission may prompt therapy. Treatment for molluscum is usually rec-ommended if lesions are in the genital area (on or near the penis, vulva, vagina, or anus). If lesions are found in this area it is a good idea to visit your healthcare provider as there is a possibility that you may have another disease spread by sexual contact. Be aware that some treatments available through the Internet may not be effective and may even be harmful.

Physical Removal

Physical removal of lesions may include cryotherapy (freezing the lesion with liquid nitro-gen), curettage (the piercing of the core and scraping of caseous or cheesy material), and laser therapy. These options are rapid and require a trained healthcare provider, may require local anesthesia, and can result in postprocedural pain, irritation, and scarring. It is not a good idea to try and remove lesions or the fluid inside of lesions yourself. By removing lesions or lesion fluid by yourself you may unintentionally autoinoculate other parts of the body or risk spread-ing it to others. By scratching or scraping the skin you could cause a bacterial infection.

Oral Therapy

Gradual removal of lesions may be achieved by oral therapy. This technique is often desir-able for pediatric patients because it is generally less painful and may be performed by parents at home in a less threatening environment. Oral cimetidine has been used as an alternative treatment for small children who are either afraid of the pain associated with cryotherapy, curettage, and laser therapy or because the possibility of scarring is to be avoided. While cimetidine is safe, painless, and well tolerated, facial mollusca do not respond as well as lesions elsewhere on the body.

Topical Therapy

Podophyllotoxin cream (0.5%) is reliable as a home therapy for men but is not recom-mended for pregnant women because of presumed toxicity to the fetus. Each lesion must be treated individually as the therapeutic effect is localized. Other options for topical therapy include iodine and salicylic acid, potassium hydroxide, tretinoin, cantharidin (a blistering agent usually applied in an office setting), and imiquimod (T cell modifier). These treatments must be prescribed by a healthcare professional.

Therapy For Immunocompromised Persons

Most therapies are effective in immunocompetent patients; however, patients with human immunodeficiency virus (HIV)/acquired immune deficiency syndrome (AIDS) or other immunosuppressing conditions often do not respond to traditional treatments. In addition, these treatments are largely ineffective in achieving long-term control in HIV patients.

Low CD4 cell counts have been linked to widespread facial mollusca and therefore have become a marker for severe HIV disease. Thus far, therapies targeted at boosting the immune system have proven the most effective therapy for molluscum contagiosum in immunocompromised persons. In extreme cases, intralesional interferon has been used to treat facial lesions in these patients. However, the severe and unpleasant side effects of interferon, such as influenza-like symptoms, site tenderness, depression, and lethargy, make it a less-than-desirable treatment. Furthermore, interferon therapy proved most effective in otherwise healthy persons. Radiation therapy is also of little benefit.

Prevention

The best way to avoid getting molluscum is by following good hygiene habits. Remember that the virus lives only in the skin and once the lesions are gone, the virus is gone and you cannot spread the virus to others.

Wash Your Hands

There are ways to prevent the spread of molluscum contagiosum. The best way is to follow good hygiene (cleanliness) habits. Keeping your hands clean is the best way to avoid molluscum infection, as well as many other infections. Hand washing removes germs that may have been picked up from other people or from surfaces that have germs on them.

Don't Scratch Or Pick At Molluscum Lesions

It is important not to touch, pick, or scratch skin that has lesions, that includes not only your own skin but anyone else's. Picking and scratching can spread the virus to other parts of the body and makes it easier to spread the disease to other people too.

Keep Molluscum Lesions Covered

It is important to keep the area with molluscum lesions clean and covered with clothing or a bandage so that others do not touch the lesions and become infected. Do remember to keep the affected skin clean and dry. Any time there is no risk of others coming into contact with your skin, such as at night when you sleep, uncover the lesions to help keep your skin healthy.

Be Careful During Sports Activities

- Do not share towels, clothing, or other personal items.

- People with molluscum should not take part in contact sports like wrestling, basketball, and football unless all lesions can be covered by clothing or bandages. Activities that use shared gear like helmets, baseball gloves and balls should also be avoided unless all lesions can be covered.

- Swimming should also be avoided unless all lesions can be covered by watertight bandages. Personal items such as towels, goggles, and swim suits should not be shared. Other items and equipment such as kick boards and water toys should be used only when all lesions are covered by clothing or watertight bandages.

Other Ways To Avoid Sharing Your Infection

- Do not shave or have electrolysis on areas with lesions.

- Don't share personal items such as unwashed clothes, hair brushes, wrist watches, and bar soap with others.

- If you have lesions on or near the penis, vulva, vagina, or anus, avoid sexual activities until you see a healthcare provider.

Long-Term Effects

Recovery from one molluscum infection does not prevent future infections. Molluscum contagiosum is not like herpes viruses which can remain dormant ("sleeping") in your body for long periods of time and then reappear. If you get new molluscum contagiosum lesions after you are cured, it means you have come in contact with an infected person or object again.

Complications

The lesions caused by molluscum are usually benign and resolve without scarring. However scratching at the lesion, or using scraping and scooping to remove the lesion, can cause scarring. For this reason, physically removing the lesion is not often recommended in otherwise healthy individuals.

The most common complication is a secondary infection caused by bacteria. Secondary infections may be a significant problem in immunocompromised patients, such as those with HIV or AIDS or those taking immunosuppressing drug therapies. In these cases, treatment to prevent further spread of the infection is recommended.

Chapter 17

Parvovirus B19 (Fifth Disease)

Fifth disease is a mild rash illness caused by parvovirus B19. This disease, also called erythema infectiosum, got its name because it was fifth in a list of historical classifications of common skin rash illnesses in children. It is more common in children than adults. A person usually gets sick with fifth disease within 4 to 14 days after getting infected with parvovirus B19.

Signs And Symptoms

The first symptoms of fifth disease are usually mild and may include:

- fever,

- runny nose, and

- headache.

Then you can get a rash on your face and body.

After several days, you may get a red rash on your face called "slapped cheek" rash. This rash is the most recognized feature of fifth disease. It is more common in children than adults.

Some people may get a second rash a few days later on their chest, back, buttocks, or arms and legs. The rash may be itchy, especially on the soles of the feet. It can vary in intensity and usually goes away in 7 to 10 days, but it can come and go for several weeks. As it starts to go away, it may look lacy.

About This Chapter: This chapter includes text excerpted from "Parvovirus B19 And Fifth Disease," Centers for Disease Control and Prevention (CDC), November 2, 2015.

You may also have painful or swollen joints.

People with fifth disease can also develop pain and swelling in their joints (polyarthropathy syndrome). This is more common in adults, especially women. Some adults with fifth disease may only have painful joints, usually in the hands, feet, or knees, and no other symptoms. The joint pain usually lasts 1 to 3 weeks, but it can last for months or longer. It usually goes away without any long-term problems.

Complications

Fifth disease is usually mild for children and adults who are otherwise healthy. But for some people fifth disease cause serious health complications.

People with weakened immune systems caused by leukemia, cancer, organ transplants, or HIV infection are at risk for serious complications from fifth disease. It can cause chronic anemia that requires medical treatment.

Transmission

Parvovirus B19—which causes fifth disease—spreads through respiratory secretions (such as saliva, sputum, or nasal mucus) when an infected person coughs or sneezes. You are most contagious when it seems like you have "just a cold" and before you get the rash or joint pain and swelling. After you get the rash you are not likely to be contagious, so then it is usually safe for you or your child to go back to work or school.

People with fifth disease who have weakened immune systems may be contagious for a longer amount of time.

Parvovirus B19 can also spread through blood or blood products. A pregnant woman who is infected with parvovirus B19 can pass the virus to her baby.

Once you recover from fifth disease, you develop immunity that generally protects you from parvovirus B19 infection in the future.

Diagnosis

Healthcare providers can often diagnose fifth disease just by seeing "slapped cheek" rash on a patient's face. A blood test can also be done to determine if you are susceptible or immune to parvovirus B19 infection or if you were recently infected. The blood test may be particularly helpful for pregnant women who may have been exposed to parvovirus B19 and are suspected to have fifth disease.

Prevention

There is no vaccine or medicine that can prevent parvovirus B19 infection. You can reduce your chance of being infected or infecting others by:

- washing your hands often with soap and water

- covering your mouth and nose when you cough or sneeze

- not touching your eyes, nose, or mouth

- avoiding close contact with people who are sick

- staying home when you are sick

After you get the rash, you are probably not contagious. So it is usually then safe for you to go back to work or for your child to return to school or a child care center.

Healthcare providers who are pregnant should know about potential risks to their baby and discuss this with their doctor.

All healthcare providers and patients should follow strict infection control practices to prevent parvovirus B19 from spreading

Treatment

Fifth disease is usually mild and will go away on its own. Children and adults who are otherwise healthy usually recover completely. Treatment usually involves relieving symptoms, such as fever, itching, and joint pain and swelling.

People who have complications from fifth disease should see their healthcare provider for medical treatment.

Chapter 18

Tinea Infections: Ringworm, Athlete's Foot, And Jock Itch

Ringworm

Ringworm is a common infection of the skin and nails that is caused by fungus. The infection is called "ringworm" because it can cause an itchy, red, circular rash. Ringworm is also called "tinea" or "dermatophytosis." The different types of ringworm are usually named for the location of the infection on the body.

Areas of the body that can be affected by ringworm include:

- Feet (tinea pedis, commonly called "athlete's foot")

- Groin, inner thighs, or buttocks (tinea cruris, commonly called "jock itch")

- Scalp (tinea capitis)

- Beard (tinea barbae)

- Hands (tinea manuum)

- Toenails or fingernails (tinea unguium, also called "onychomycosis") Click here for more information about fungal nail infections. Note: please link this last sentence to the new nail infections page.

- Other parts of the body such as arms or legs (tinea corporis)

About This Chapter: Text under the heading "Ringworm" is excerpted from "Fungal Diseases—Ringworm," Centers for Disease Control and Prevention (CDC), December 4, 2015; Text under the heading "Athlete's Foot (Tinea Pedis)" is excerpted from "Hygiene-Related Diseases," Centers for Disease Control and Prevention (CDC), February 6, 2017; Text under the heading "Jock Itch" is © 2018 Omnigraphics. Reviewed August 2017.

Approximately 40 different species of fungi can cause ringworm; the scientific names for the types of fungi that cause ringworm are *Trichophyton*, *Microsporum*, and *Epidermophyton*.

Symptoms

Ringworm can affect skin on almost any part of the body as well as fingernails and toenails. The symptoms of ringworm often depend on which part of the body is infected, but they generally include:

- Itchy skin

- Ring-shaped rash

- Red, scaly, cracked skin

- Hair loss

Symptoms typically appear between 4 and 14 days after the skin comes in contact with the fungi that cause ringworm.

Symptoms Of Ringworm By Location On The Body

- **Feet (tinea pedis or "athlete's foot"):** The symptoms of ringworm on the feet include red, swollen, peeling, itchy skin between the toes (especially between the pinky toe and the one next to it). The sole and heel of the foot may also be affected. In severe cases, the skin on the feet can blister.

- **Scalp (tinea capitis):** Ringworm on the scalp usually looks like a scaly, itchy, red, circular bald spot. The bald spot can grow in size and multiple spots might develop if the infection spreads. Ringworm on the scalp is more common in children than it is in adults.

- **Groin (tinea cruris or "jock itch"):** Ringworm on the groin looks like scaly, itchy, red spots, usually on the inner sides of the skin folds of the thigh.

- **Beard (tinea barbae):** Symptoms of ringworm on the beard include scaly, itchy, red spots on the cheeks, chin, and upper neck. The spots might become crusted over or filled with pus, and the affected hair might fall out.

Ringworm Risk And Prevention

Who Gets Ringworm?

Ringworm is very common. Anyone can get ringworm, but people who have weakened immune systems may be especially at risk for infection and may have problems fighting off a ringworm infection. People who use public showers or locker rooms, athletes (particularly those who are involved in contact sports such as wrestling), people who wear tight shoes and have excessive sweating, and people who have close contact with animals may also be more likely to come in contact with the fungi that cause ringworm.

How Can I Prevent Ringworm?

- Keep your skin clean and dry.

- Wear shoes that allow air to circulate freely around your feet.

- Don't walk barefoot in areas like locker rooms or public showers.

- Clip your fingernails and toenails short and keep them clean.

- Change your socks and underwear at least once a day.

- Don't share clothing, towels, sheets, or other personal items with someone who has ringworm.

- Wash your hands with soap and running water after playing with pets. If you suspect that your pet has ringworm, take it to see a veterinarian. If your pet has ringworm, follow the steps below to prevent spreading the infection.

- If you're an athlete involved in close contact sports, shower immediately after your practice session or match, and keep all of your sports gear and uniform clean. Don't share sports gear (helmet, etc.) with other players.

Sources Of Infection

The fungi that cause ringworm can live on skin and in the environment. There are three main ways that ringworm can spread:

1. From a person who has ringworm.

   People can get ringworm after contact with someone who has the infection. To avoid spreading the infection, people with ringworm shouldn't share clothing, towels, combs, or other personal items with other people.

2. From an animal that has ringworm.

   People can get ringworm after touching an animal that has ringworm. Many different kinds of animals can spread ringworm to people, including dogs and cats, especially kittens and puppies. Other animals, like cows, goats, pigs, and horses can also spread ringworm to people.

3. From the environment.

The fungi that cause ringworm can live on surfaces, particularly in damp areas like locker rooms and public showers. For that reason, it's a good idea not to walk barefoot in these places.

Diagnosis

Your healthcare provider can usually diagnose ringworm by looking at the affected skin and asking questions about your symptoms. He or she may also take a small skin scraping to be examined under a microscope or sent to a laboratory for a fungal culture.

Physical examination

A thorough history and physical examination is often sufficient to diagnose tinea. The classic lesion is an erythematous, raised, scaly ring with central clearing. Multiple lesions may be present. The severity of the infection can range from mild, scaly lesions, to erythematous, exudative lesions characteristic of superimposed bacterial infections.

Microscopy

Potassium hydroxide (KOH) stain a commonly-used method for diagnosing tinea because it is inexpensive, easy to perform, and has high sensitivity. Scrapings from the lesion(s) are placed in a drop of KOH and examined under a microscope for the presence of fungal hyphae.

Ultraviolet light (Wood's lamp)

Normally, ultraviolet light is not useful in the diagnosis of tinea with the exception of two species—*Microsporum canis* and *audouinii*. Although both species fluoresce blue-green under a Wood's lamp, both species are uncommon causes of tinea infections. A Wood's lamp may be useful to differentiate between erythrasma caused by *Corynebacterium minutissimum* (which fluoresces coal-red) from tinea cruris, which is nonfluorescent.

Culture

Fungal culture can be performed as a confirmatory test if results from a KOH stain are inconclusive. Hair and/or scrapings extracted from affected areas are placed on Sabouraud's medium. Fungal culture is more specific than KOH stain, but it can take up to three weeks to become positive.

Treatment

The treatment for ringworm depends on its location on the body and how serious the infection is. Some forms of ringworm can be treated with nonprescription ("over-the-counter") medications, but other forms of ringworm need treatment with prescription antifungal medication.

- Ringworm on the skin like athlete's foot (tinea pedis) and jock itch (tinea cruris) can usually be treated with nonprescription antifungal creams, lotions, or powders applied to the skin for 2 to 4 weeks. There are many nonprescription products available to treat ringworm, including:

    - Clotrimazole (Lotrimin, Mycelex)

    - Miconazole (Aloe Vesta Antifungal, Azolen, Baza Antifungal, Carrington Antifungal, Critic Aid Clear, Cruex Prescription Strength, DermaFungal, Desenex, Fungoid Tincture, Micaderm, Micatin, Micro-Guard, Miranel, Mitrazol, Podactin, Remedy Antifungal, Secura Antifungal)

    - Terbinafine (Lamisil)

    - Ketoconazole (Xolegel)

For nonprescription creams, lotions, or powders, follow the directions on the package label. Contact your healthcare provider if your infection doesn't go away or gets worse.

- Ringworm on the scalp (tinea capitis) usually needs to be treated with prescription antifungal medication taken by mouth for 1 to 3 months. Creams, lotions, or powders don't work for ringworm on the scalp. Prescription antifungal medications used to treat ringworm on the scalp include:
    - Griseofulvin (Grifulvin V, Gris-PEG)
    - Terbinafine
    - Itraconazole (Onmel, Sporanox)
    - Fluconazole (Diflucan)

You should contact your healthcare provider if:

- Your infection gets worse or doesn't go away after using nonprescription medications.
- You or your child has ringworm on the scalp. Ringworm on the scalp needs to be treated with prescription antifungal medication.

Athlete's Foot (Tinea Pedis)

Athlete's foot, or *tinea pedis*, is an infection of the skin and feet that can be caused by a variety of different fungi. Although *tinea pedis* can affect any portion of the foot, the infection most often affects the space between the toes. Athlete's foot is typically characterized by skin fissures or scales that can be red and itchy.

Tinea pedis is spread through contact with infected skin scales or contact with fungi in damp areas (for example, showers, locker rooms, swimming pools). *Tinea pedis* can be a chronic infection that recurs frequently. Treatment may include topical creams (applied to the surface of the skin) or oral medications.

Appropriate hygiene techniques may help to prevent or control *tinea pedis*. The following hygiene techniques should be followed:

Prevention of athlete's foot:

- Nails should be clipped short and kept clean. Nails can house and spread the infection.

- Avoid walking barefoot in locker rooms or public showers (wear sandals).

For control of athlete's foot infection, persons with active tinea pedis infection should:

- Keep feet clean, dry, and cool.

- Avoid using swimming pools, public showers, or foot baths.

- Wear sandals when possible or air shoes out by alternating them every 2–3 days.

- Avoid wearing closed shoes and wearing socks made from fabric that doesn't dry easily (for example, nylon).

- Treat the infection with recommended medication.

Jock Itch

Jock itch (tinea cruris) is a fungal skin infection affecting the genital area, inner thighs, and buttocks. It is characterized by an itchy, ring-shaped rash in moist areas of the skin. It is caused by the same fungus that causes athlete's foot. The fungus spreads from the foot to the groin by touch or through contaminated towels or clothing from person to person.

Jock itch is named so because it is seen in people who sweat a lot, which is common in athletes. It is also seen in people who are overweight.

Jock itch is usually diagnosed with a physical examination or with a laboratory culture test in unclear cases. Though uncomfortable, jock itch is not a serious complaint and it can be treated with the application of topical antifungal medications for one to two weeks.

Jock itch can be prevented by staying dry, wearing clean and fitting clothes, and avoiding sharing personal items such as towels, clothes, etc.

Reference

"Jock Itch," Mayo Foundation for Medical Education and Research (MFMER), July 26, 2016.

Chapter 19

Scabies

What Is Scabies?

Scabies is an infestation of the skin by the human itch mite *(Sarcoptes scabiei var. hominis)*. The microscopic scabies mite burrows into the upper layer of the skin where it lives and lays its eggs. The most common symptoms of scabies are intense itching and a pimple-like skin rash. The scabies mite usually is spread by direct, prolonged, skin-to-skin contact with a person who has scabies.

Scabies is found worldwide and affects people of all races and social classes. Scabies can spread rapidly under crowded conditions where close body and skin contact is frequent. Institutions such as nursing homes, extended-care facilities, and prisons are often sites of scabies outbreaks. Child care facilities also are a common site of scabies infestations.

What Is Crusted (Norwegian) Scabies?

Crusted scabies is a severe form of scabies that can occur in some persons who are immunocompromised (have a weak immune system), elderly, disabled, or debilitated. It is also called Norwegian scabies. Persons with crusted scabies have thick crusts of skin that contain large numbers of scabies mites and eggs. Persons with crusted scabies are very contagious to other persons and can spread the infestation easily both by direct skin-to-skin contact and by contamination of items such as their clothing, bedding, and furniture. Persons with crusted scabies may not show the usually signs and symptoms of scabies such as the characteristic rash or

About This Chapter: This chapter includes text excerpted from "Scabies—Scabies Frequently Asked Questions (FAQs)," Centers for Disease Control and Prevention (CDC), November 2, 2010. Reviewed August 2017.

itching (pruritus). Persons with crusted scabies should receive quick and aggressive medical treatment for their infestation to prevent outbreaks of scabies.

How Soon After Infestation Do Symptoms Of Scabies Begin?

If a person has never had scabies before, symptoms may take as long as 4–6 weeks to begin. It is important to remember that an infested person can spread scabies during this time, even if he/she does not have symptoms yet.

In a person who has had scabies before, symptoms usually appear much sooner (1–4 days) after exposure.

What Are The Signs And Symptoms Of Scabies Infestation?

The most common signs and symptoms of scabies are intense itching (pruritus), especially at night, and a pimple-like (papular) itchy rash. The itching and rash each may affect much of the body or be limited to common sites such as the wrist, elbow, armpit, webbing between the fingers, nipple, penis, waist, belt-line, and buttocks. The rash also can include tiny blisters (vesicles) and scales. Scratching the rash can cause skin sores; sometimes these sores become infected by bacteria.

Tiny burrows sometimes are seen on the skin; these are caused by the female scabies mite tunneling just beneath the surface of the skin. These burrows appear as tiny raised and crooked (serpiginous) grayish-white or skin-colored lines on the skin surface. Because mites are often few in number (only 10–15 mites per person), these burrows may be difficult to find. They are found most often in the webbing between the fingers, in the skin folds on the wrist, elbow, or knee, and on the penis, breast, or shoulder blades.

The head, face, neck, palms, and soles often are involved in infants and very young children, but usually not adults and older children.

Persons with crusted scabies may not show the usual signs and symptoms of scabies such as the characteristic rash or itching (pruritus).

How Did I Get Scabies?

Scabies usually is spread by direct, prolonged, skin-to-skin contact with a person who has scabies. Contact generally must be prolonged; a quick handshake or hug usually will not spread scabies. Scabies is spread easily to sexual partners and household members. Scabies in adults frequently is sexually acquired. Scabies sometimes is spread indirectly by sharing articles such as clothing, towels, or bedding used by an infested person; however, such indirect spread can occur much more easily when the infested person has crusted scabies.

How Is Scabies Infestation Diagnosed?

Diagnosis of a scabies infestation usually is made based on the customary appearance and distribution of the rash and the presence of burrows. Whenever possible, the diagnosis of scabies should be confirmed by identifying the mite, mite eggs, or mite fecal matter (scybala). This can be done by carefully removing a mite from the end of its burrow using the tip of a needle or by obtaining skin scraping to examine under a microscope for mites, eggs, or mite fecal matter. It is important to remember that a person can still be infested even if mites, eggs, or fecal matter cannot be found; typically fewer than 10–15 mites can be present on the entire body of an infested person who is otherwise healthy. However, persons with crusted scabies can be infested with thousands of mites and should be considered highly contagious.

How Long Can Scabies Mites Live?

On a person, scabies mites can live for as long as 1–2 months. Off a person, scabies mites usually do not survive more than 48–72 hours. Scabies mites will die if exposed to a temperature of 50°C (122°F) for 10 minutes.

Can Scabies Be Treated?

Yes. Products used to treat scabies are called scabicides because they kill scabies mites; some also kill eggs. Scabicides to treat human scabies are available only with a doctor's prescription; no "over-the-counter" (nonprescription) products have been tested and approved for humans.

Always follow carefully the instructions provided by the doctor and pharmacist, as well as those contained in the box or printed on the label. When treating adults and older children, scabicide cream or lotion is applied to all areas of the body from the neck down to the feet and toes; when treating infants and young children, the cream or lotion also is applied to the head and neck. The medication should be left on the body for the recommended time before it is washed off. Clean clothes should be worn after treatment.

In addition to the infested person, treatment also is recommended for household members and sexual contacts, particularly those who have had prolonged skin-to-skin contact with the infested person. All persons should be treated at the same time in order to prevent reinfestation.

Retreatment may be necessary if itching continues more than 2–4 weeks after treatment or if new burrows or rash continue to appear.

Never use a scabicide intended for veterinary or agricultural use to treat humans!

Who Should Be Treated For Scabies?

Anyone who is diagnosed with scabies, as well as his or her sexual partners and other contacts who have had prolonged skin-to-skin contact with the infested person, should be treated. Treatment is recommended for members of the same household as the person with scabies, particularly those persons who have had prolonged skin-to-skin contact with the infested person. All persons should be treated at the same time to prevent reinfestation.

Retreatment may be necessary if itching continues more than 2–4 weeks after treatment or if new burrows or rash continue to appear.

How Soon After Treatment Will I Feel Better?

If itching continues more than 2–4 weeks after initial treatment or if new burrows or rash continue to appear (if initial treatment includes more than one application or dose, then the 2–4 time period begins after the last application or dose), retreatment with scabicide may be necessary; seek the advice of a physician.

Did I Get Scabies From My Pet?

No. Animals do not spread human scabies. Pets can become infested with a different kind of scabies mite that does not survive or reproduce on humans but causes "mange" in animals. If an animal with "mange" has close contact with a person, the animal mite can get under the person's skin and cause temporary itching and skin irritation. However, the animal mite cannot reproduce on a person and will die on its own in a couple of days. Although the person does not need to be treated, the animal should be treated because its mites can continue to burrow into the person's skin and cause symptoms until the animal has been treated successfully.

Can Scabies Be Spread By Swimming In A Public Pool?

Scabies is spread by prolonged skin-to-skin contact with a person who has scabies. Scabies sometimes also can be spread by contact with items such as clothing, bedding, or towels that have been used by a person with scabies, but such spread is very uncommon unless the infested person has crusted scabies.

Scabies is very unlikely to be spread by water in a swimming pool. Except for a person with crusted scabies, only about 10–15 scabies mites are present on an infested person; it is extremely unlikely that any would emerge from under wet skin.

Although uncommon, scabies can be spread by sharing a towel or item of clothing that has been used by a person with scabies.

How Can I Remove Scabies Mites From My House Or Carpet?

Scabies mites do not survive more than 2–3 days away from human skin. Items such as bedding, clothing, and towels used by a person with scabies can be decontaminated by machine-washing in hot water and drying using the hot cycle or by dry-cleaning. Items that cannot be washed or dry-cleaned can be decontaminated by removing from any body contact for at least 72 hours.

Because persons with crusted scabies are considered very infectious, careful vacuuming of furniture and carpets in rooms used by these persons is recommended.

Fumigation of living areas is unnecessary.

How Can I Remove Scabies Mites From My Clothes?

Scabies mites do not survive more than 2–3 days away from human skin. Items such as bedding, clothing, and towels used by a person with scabies can be decontaminated by machine-washing in hot water and drying using the hot cycle or by dry-cleaning. Items that cannot be washed or dry-cleaned can be decontaminated by removing from any body contact for at least 72 hours.

If I Come In Contact With A Person Who Has Scabies, Should I Treat Myself?

No. If a person thinks he or she might have scabies, he/she should contact a doctor. The doctor can examine the person, confirm the diagnosis of scabies, and prescribe an appropriate treatment. Products used to treat scabies in humans are available only with a doctor's prescription.

Sleeping with or having sex with any scabies infested person presents a high risk for transmission. The longer a person has skin-to-skin exposure, the greater is the likelihood for transmission to occur. Although briefly shaking hands with a person who has noncrusted scabies could be considered as presenting a relatively low risk, holding the hand of a person with scabies for 5–10 minutes could be considered to present a relatively high risk of transmission. However, transmission can occur even after brief skin-to-skin contact, such as a handshake, with a person who has crusted scabies. In general, a person who has skin-to-skin contact with a person who has crusted scabies would be considered a good candidate for treatment.

To determine when prophylactic treatment should be given to reduce the risk of transmission, early consultation should be sought with a healthcare provider who understands:

1. The type of scabies (i.e., noncrusted vs crusted) to which a person has been exposed;

2. The degree and duration of skin exposure that a person has had to the infested patient;

3. Whether the exposure occurred before or after the patient was treated for scabies; and,

4. Whether the exposed person works in an environment where he/she would be likely to expose other people during the asymptomatic incubation period. For example, a nurse or caretaker who works in a nursing home or hospital often would be treated prophylactically to reduce the risk of further scabies transmission in the facility.

Chapter 20

Swimmer's Itch

What Is Swimmer's Itch?

Swimmer's itch, also called cercarial dermatitis, appears as a skin rash caused by an allergic reaction to certain microscopic parasites that infect some birds and mammals. These parasites are released from infected snails into fresh and salt water (such as lakes, ponds, and oceans). While the parasite's preferred host is the specific bird or mammal, if the parasite comes into contact with a swimmer, it burrows into the skin causing an allergic reaction and rash. Swimmer's itch is found throughout the world and is more frequent during summer months.

How Does Water Become Infested With The Parasite?

The adult parasite lives in the blood of infected animals such as ducks, geese, gulls, swans, and certain mammals such as muskrats and raccoons. The parasites produce eggs that are passed in the feces of infected birds or mammals.

If the eggs land in or are washed into the water, the eggs hatch, releasing small, free-swimming microscopic larvae. These larvae swim in the water in search of a certain species of aquatic snail.

If the larvae find one of these snails, they infect the snail, multiply and undergo further development. Infected snails release a different type of microscopic larvae (or cercariae, hence the name cercarial dermatitis) into the water. This larval form then swims about

About This Chapter: This chapter includes text excerpted from "Swimmer's Itch—Swimmer's Itch FAQs," Centers for Disease Control and Prevention (CDC), January 10, 2012. Reviewed August 2017.

searching for a suitable host (bird, muskrat) to continue the lifecycle. Although humans are not suitable hosts, the microscopic larvae burrow into the swimmer's skin, and may cause an allergic reaction and rash. Because these larvae cannot develop inside a human, they soon die.

What Are The Signs And Symptoms Of Swimmer's Itch?

Symptoms of swimmer's itch may include:

- tingling, burning, or itching of the skin

- small reddish pimples

- small blisters

Within minutes to days after swimming in contaminated water, you may experience tingling, burning, or itching of the skin. Small reddish pimples appear within twelve hours. Pimples may develop into small blisters. Scratching the areas may result in secondary bacterial infections. Itching may last up to a week or more, but will gradually go away.

Because swimmer's itch is caused by an allergic reaction to infection, the more often you swim or wade in contaminated water, the more likely you are to develop more serious symptoms. The greater the number of exposures to contaminated water, the more intense and immediate symptoms of swimmer's itch will be.

Be aware that swimmer's itch is not the only rash that may occur after swimming in fresh or salt water.

Do I Need To See My Healthcare Provider For Treatment?

Most cases of swimmer's itch do not require medical attention. If you have a rash, you may try the following for relief:

- Use corticosteroid cream

- Apply cool compresses to the affected areas

- Bathe in Epsom salts or baking soda

- Soak in colloidal oatmeal baths

- Apply baking soda paste to the rash (made by stirring water into baking soda until it reaches a paste-like consistency)

- Use an anti-itch lotion

Though difficult, try not to scratch. Scratching may cause the rash to become infected. If itching is severe, your healthcare provider may suggest prescription-strength lotions or creams to lessen your symptoms.

Can Swimmer's Itch Be Spread From Person-To-Person?

Swimmer's itch is not contagious and cannot be spread from one person to another.

Who Is At Risk For Swimmer's Itch?

Anyone who swims or wades in infested water may be at risk. Larvae are more likely to be present in shallow water by the shoreline. Children are most often affected because they tend to swim, wade, and play in the shallow water more than adults. Also, they are less likely to towel dry themselves when leaving the water.

Once An Outbreak Of Swimmer's Itch Has Occurred In Water, Will The Water Always Be Unsafe?

No. Many factors must be present for swimmer's itch to become a problem in water. Since these factors change (sometimes within a swim season), swimmer's itch will not always be a problem. However, there is no way to know how long water may be unsafe. Larvae generally survive for 24 hours once they are released from the snail. However, an infected snail will continue to produce cercariae throughout the remainder of its life. For future snails to become infected, migratory birds or mammals in the area must also be infected so the life-cycle can continue.

Is It Safe To Swim In My Swimming Pool?

Yes. As long as your swimming pool is well maintained and chlorinated, there is no risk of swimmer's itch. The appropriate snails must be present in order for swimmer's itch to occur.

What Can Be Done To Reduce The Risk Of Swimmer's Itch?

To reduce the likelihood of developing swimmer's itch:

- Do not swim in areas where swimmer's itch is a known problem or where signs have been posted warning of unsafe water.

- Do not swim near or wade in marshy areas where snails are commonly found.

- Towel dry or shower immediately after leaving the water.

- Do not attract birds (e.g., by feeding them) to areas where people are swimming.

- Encourage health officials to post signs on shorelines where swimmer's itch is a current problem.

Chapter 21

Fungal Nail Infections

Fungal nail infections are common infections of the fingernails or toenails that can cause the nail to become discolored, thick, and more likely to crack and break. Infections are more common in toenails than fingernails. The technical name for a fungal nail infection is "onychomycosis."

Symptoms

Nails with a fungal infection are often:

- Discolored (yellow, brown, or white)

- Thick

- Fragile or cracked

A fungal nail infection usually isn't painful unless it becomes severe.

Some people who have fungal toenail infections also have a fungal skin infection on the foot, especially between the toes (commonly called "athlete's foot").

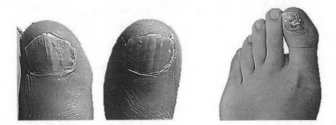

Figure 21.1. Fungal Nail Infections

About This Chapter: This chapter includes text excerpted from "Fungal Nail Infections," Centers for Disease Control and Prevention (CDC), January 25, 2017.

How Does Someone Get A Fungal Nail Infection?

Fungal nail infections can be caused by many different types of fungi (yeasts or molds) that live in the environment. Small cracks in your nail or the surrounding skin can allow these germs to enter your nail and cause an infection.

Who Gets Fungal Nail Infections?

Anyone can get a fungal nail infection. Some people may be more likely than others to get a fungal nail infection, including older adults and people who have the following conditions:

- A nail injury or nail surgery
- Diabetes
- A weakened immune system
- Blood circulation problems
- Athlete's foot (ringworm on the foot)

Prevention

- Keep your hands and feet clean and dry.
- Clip your fingernails and toenails short and keep them clean.
- Don't walk barefoot in areas like locker rooms or public showers.
- Don't share nail clippers with other people.
- When visiting a nail salon, choose a salon that is clean and licensed by your state's cosmetology board. Make sure the salon sterilizes its instruments (nail clippers, scissors, etc.) after each use, or, you can bring your own.

Diagnosis

Your healthcare provider may diagnose a fungal nail infection by looking at the affected nail and asking questions about your symptoms. He or she may also take a nail clipping to look at under a microscope or send to a laboratory for a fungal culture.

Treatment

Fungal nail infections can be difficult to cure, and they typically don't go away without antifungal treatment. The best treatment for a fungal nail infection is usually prescription anti-fungal pills taken by mouth. In severe cases, a doctor might remove the nail completely. It can take several months to a year for the infection to go away.

Part Four
Other Diseases And Disorders Affecting The Skin

Chapter 22

Albinism

Albinism is a group of inherited disorders that results in little or no production of the pigment melanin, which determines the color of the skin, hair and eyes. Melanin also plays a role in the development of certain optical nerves, so all forms of albinism cause problems with the development and function of the eyes. Other symptoms can include light skin or changes in skin color; very white to brown hair; very light blue to brown eye color that may appear red in some light and may change with age; sensitivity to sun exposure; and increased risk of developing skin cancer. Albinism is caused by mutations in one of several genes, and most types are inherited in an autosomal recessive manner. Although there's no cure, people with the disorder can take steps to improve vision and avoid too much sun exposure.

Inheritance

Different types of albinism can have different patterns of inheritance, depending on the genetic cause of the condition. Oculocutaneous albinism (OCA) involves the eyes, hair, and skin. Ocular albinism (OA), which is much less common, involves primarily the eyes, while skin and hair may appear similar or slightly lighter than that of other family members. Mutations in several different genes, on different chromosomes, can cause different types of albinism.

OCA is inherited in an autosomal recessive manner. This means that two mutations are necessary for an individual to have OCA. Individuals normally have two copies of each numbered chromosome and the genes on them—one inherited from the father, the other inherited

About This Chapter: This chapter includes text excerpted from "Albinism," Genetic and Rare Diseases Information Center (GARD), National Center for Advancing Translational Sciences (NCATS), May 24, 2016.

from the mother. Neither of these gene copies is functional in people with albinism. Each unaffected parent of an individual with an autosomal recessive condition carries one functional copy of the causative gene and one nonfunctional copy. They are referred to as carriers, and do not typically show signs or symptoms of the condition. Both parents must carry a defective OCA gene to have a child with albinism. When two individuals who are carriers for the same autosomal recessive condition have children, with each pregnancy there is a 25 percent (1 in 4) risk for the child to have the condition, a 50 percent (1 in 2) risk for the child to be an unaffected carrier like each of the parents, and a 25 percent chance for the child to not have the condition and not be a carrier.

Ocular albinism type 1 is inherited in an X-linked pattern. A condition is considered X-linked if the mutated gene that causes the disorder is located on the X chromosome, one of the two sex chromosomes. In males (who have only one X chromosome and one Y), one altered copy of the causative gene in each cell is sufficient to cause the characteristic features of ocular albinism, because males do not have another X chromosome with a working copy of the gene. Because females have two copies of the X chromosome, women with only one copy of a mutation in each cell usually do not experience vision loss or other significant eye abnormalities. They may have mild changes in retinal pigmentation that can be detected during an eye examination.

Researchers have also identified several other genes in which mutations can result in albinism with other features. One group of these includes at least nine genes (on different chromosomes) leading to Hermansky-Pudlak Syndrome (HPS). In addition to albinism, HPS is associated with bleeding problems and bruising. Some forms are also associated with lung and bowel disease. Like OCA, HPS is inherited in an autosomal recessive manner.

Treatment

The goal of treatment is to address the symptoms present in each individual. People with albinism should protect their skin and eyes from the sun. This can be done by:

- avoiding prolonged exposure to the sun,

- using sunscreen with a high sun-protection factor (SPF) rating (20 or higher),

- covering up completely with clothing when exposed to the sun, and

- wearing sunglasses with ultraviolet (UV) protection.

Individuals with vision problems may need corrective lenses. They should also have regular follow-up exams with an ophthalmologist. In rare cases, surgery may be needed. Individuals with albinism should also have regular skin assessments to screen for skin cancer or lesions that can lead to cancer.

Prognosis

Most people with albinism live a normal life span and have the same types of medical problems as the rest of the population. Although the risk to develop skin cancer is increased, with careful surveillance and prompt treatment, this is usually curable.

Chapter 23

Birthmarks And Giant Congenital Melanocytic Nevus

What Are Birthmarks?

Birthmarks are abnormalities of the skin that are present when a baby is born. There are two types of birthmarks.

- Vascular birthmarks are made up of blood vessels that haven't formed correctly. They are usually red. Two types of vascular birthmarks are hemangiomas and port-wine stains.

- Pigmented birthmarks are made of a cluster of pigment cells which cause color in skin. They can be many different colors, from tan to brown, gray to black, or even blue. Moles can be birthmarks.

No one knows what causes many types of birthmarks, but some run in families. Your baby's doctor will look at the birthmark to see if it needs any treatment or if it should be watched. Pigmented birthmarks aren't usually treated, except for moles. Treatment for vascular birthmarks includes laser surgery.

Most birthmarks are not serious, and some go away on their own. Some stay the same or get worse as you get older. Usually birthmarks are only a concern for your appearance. But certain types can increase your risk of skin cancer. If your birthmark bleeds, hurts, itches, or becomes infected, call your healthcare provider.

About This Chapter: Text under the heading "What Are Birthmarks?" is excerpted from "Birthmarks," MedlinePlus, National Institutes of Health (NIH), April 18, 2016; Text under the heading "What Is Giant Congenital Melanocytic Nevus?" is excerpted from "Giant Congenital Melanocytic Nevus," Genetics Home Reference (GHR), National Institutes of Health (NIH), December 2014.

What Is Giant Congenital Melanocytic Nevus?

Giant congenital melanocytic nevus is a skin condition characterized by an abnormally dark, noncancerous skin patch (nevus) that is composed of pigment-producing cells called melanocytes. It is present from birth (congenital) or is noticeable soon after birth. The nevus may be small in infants, but it will usually grow at the same rate the body grows and will eventually be at least 40 cm (15.75 inches) across. The nevus can appear anywhere on the body, but it is more often found on the trunk or limbs. The color ranges from tan to black and can become darker or lighter over time. The surface of a nevus can be flat, rough, raised, thickened, or bumpy; the surface can vary in different regions of the nevus, and it can change over time. The skin of the nevus is often dry and prone to irritation and itching (dermatitis). Excessive hair growth (hypertrichosis) can occur within the nevus. There is often less fat tissue under the skin of the nevus; the skin may appear thinner there than over other areas of the body.

People with giant congenital melanocytic nevus may have more than one nevus (plural: nevi). The other nevi are often smaller than the giant nevus. Affected individuals may have one or two additional nevi or multiple small nevi that are scattered over the skin; these are known as satellite or disseminated nevi.

Affected individuals may feel anxiety or emotional stress due to the impact the nevus may have on their appearance and their health. Children with giant congenital melanocytic nevus can develop emotional or behavior problems.

Some people with giant congenital melanocytic nevus develop a condition called neurocutaneous melanosis, which is the presence of pigment-producing skin cells (melanocytes) in the tissue that covers the brain and spinal cord. These melanocytes may be spread out or grouped together in clusters. Their growth can cause increased pressure in the brain, leading to headache, vomiting, irritability, seizures, and movement problems. Tumors in the brain may also develop.

Individuals with giant congenital melanocytic nevus have an increased risk of developing an aggressive form of cancer called melanoma, which arises from melanocytes. Estimates vary, but it is generally thought that people with giant congenital melanocytic nevus have a 5 to 10 percent lifetime risk of developing melanoma. Melanoma commonly begins in the nevus, but it can develop when melanocytes that invade other tissues, such as those in the brain and spinal cord, become cancerous. When melanoma occurs in people with giant congenital melanocytic nevus, the survival rate is low.

Other types of tumors can also develop in individuals with giant congenital melanocytic nevus, including soft tissue tumors (sarcomas), fatty tumors (lipomas), and tumors of the nerve cells (schwannomas).

Chapter 24

Cellulite And Stretch Marks

What Is Cellulite?

Cellulite is the term for the dimpled, lumpy appearance of flesh caused by fat deposits just beneath the skin. Cellulite is more common in women than in men and generally appears where fat is normally distributed on women, such as the buttocks, thighs, hips, and abdomen. It is not a serious condition, and medical professionals consider it to be a normal part of a person's appearance.

What Does Cellulite Look Like?

Cellulite is often compared to cottage cheese or the peel of an orange. Mild cellulite can be seen only if the skin is pinched where it is present. In severe cases of cellulite, the skin may appear extremely creased or rumpled.

What Causes Cellulite?

Researchers do not know the exact cause of cellulite, but they believe the condition has to do with the collagen fibers that bring together the skin and the layer of fat just underneath it. Those fibers can stretch, break, or become tight, causing the fat to swell out and push against the skin, creating a lumpy appearance.

Genetics likely play a role in how visible cellulite is and where it appears. Both lean and overweight individuals can have cellulite, but the condition is more visible with weight gain. The condition generally makes its first appearance after puberty, but it may also develop as people age as the skin loses elasticity.

"Cellulite And Stretch Marks," © 2018 Omnigraphics. Reviewed August 2017.

Other factors affect the appearance of cellulite, including:

- Hormonal changes

- Poor metabolism (how efficiently your body burns fuel)

- Poor diet

- Fad dieting or yo-yo dieting where you quickly lose and gain back weight

- Smoking

- Sedentary lifestyle

How Is Cellulite Treated?

Since health professionals consider the condition normal, any treatment is cosmetic, or focused on lessening the appearance of cellulite. An array of commercial creams, nutrition supplements, and procedures claiming to "cure" or minimize cellulite are available, but none are scientifically proven or consistently effective. Many also have side effects, including skin irritation, infection, and unevenness.

The following medical procedures can be used by doctors to minimize the appearance of cellulite, but none are permanent and carry some risk:

- **Cryolipolysis:** A noninvasive procedure that removes fat deposits in the abdomen and the sides of the body by freezing lipids in fat cells.

- **Lasers and radiofrequency systems:** Classified into three systems: one combines radio-frequency technology, infrared light, and tissue massage for treatment; the second system combines tissue massage and diode laser; and the third system uses radio frequency.

- **Liposuction:** A procedure in which a surgeon inserts a tube into tiny incisions to suction away fat cells, liposuction periodically used to minimize cellulite. However, the procedure is not generally recommended since, while it can reshape the body, it can often make cellulite appear worse.

Tips That Can Help Avoid Cellulite

Knowing that cellulite is normal and maintaining a healthy body image is key to "living with" it. Also, pursuing habits that keep your body healthy can help minimize the appearance of cellulite, including:

- Regular exercise

- Eating right

- Staying hydrated
- Maintaining a healthy weight
- Quitting smoking or not starting

What Are Stretch Marks?

Stretch marks are streaks that often appear like lines or stripes and are caused by stretching of the skin. Stretch marks are usually seen in the abdomen, hips, thighs, and buttocks, and the breasts in women. They are harmless and painless, and they often fade over time.

What Do Stretch Marks Look Like?

Stretch marks look like lines, stripes, or bands on different areas of the skin. They may vary in how they look depending on how long they have existed, their location on the body, and what color skin an individual has. Stretch marks can be pink, purple, red, or blue lines covering large portions of the skin on the pelvic regions. Over a period of time, the stretch marks may become whitish in color and look similar to scars.

What Causes Stretch Marks?

Anyone can get stretch marks and the stretching of skin that leads to them can have a variety of causes. In teens, growth spurts during in puberty can cause stretch marks. Excessive weight gain, pregnancy, and some genetic disorders such as Cushing syndrome (a high level of hormone cortisol in the body) and Ehlers-Danlos syndrome (EDS) can cause stretch marks. You can also be at greater risk for having stretch marks if members of your family have had them as well.

Should Stretch Marks Be Treated?

Since stretch marks are harmless and often fade over time, treatment is unnecessary. However, if you are particularly self-conscious about their appearance, you can talk to your doctor about cosmetic treatments that include retinoid creams, laser treatments, and microdermabrasion. None of these treatments are completely proven to be effective and should be weighed against the how much the treatment costs and how much time it will take.

References

1. "Cellulite," National Institutes of Health (NIH), December 10, 2016.
2. "Can You Beat Cellulite?" Web MD, n.d.

3. "Cellulite," Mayo Clinic, n.d.

4. "Stretch Marks," National Institutes of Health (NIH), April 14, 2015.

5. "Stretch Marks," Mayo Clinic, n.d.

Chapter 25

Cysts: Epidermoid (Sebaceous), Pilonidal, And Lipoma

Cysts

Cysts are sac- or capsule-like structures filled with fluid, semisolid, or gaseous substances, depending on where the cyst is found. Cysts are not cancerous and can develop in the skin, lungs, kidneys, ovaries, and other parts of the body. Cysts in the skin grow slowly and feel like smooth bumps when you touch them. They generally do not cause symptoms unless they are infected or impinge on a nerve or blood vessel.

Epidermoid Cysts

Cysts found in the skin are commonly epidermoid cysts, noncancerous bumps that appear on the face, neck, and chest. Epidermoid cysts grow slowly and are usually painless. They generally do not require treatment unless they get infected, cause pain, or you considered their appearance to be unattractive.

Causes Of Epidermoid Cysts

The skin is made in part of a thin layer of protective cells that sheds continuously. Sometimes, these cells move inwards and multiply rather than slough away. These cells eventually turn into epidermoid cysts. Epidermoid cysts sometimes form due to injury or irritation to the skin or part of a hair follicle.

Symptoms Of Epidermoid Cysts

Symptoms of epidermoid cysts include:

- A small bump in the skin, face, neck, or chest
- A blackhead that plugs the center opening of the cyst
- A thick, yellow substance that drains from the cyst
- Swelling, redness, and tenderness if the cyst is infected

Diagnosis Of Epidermoid Cysts

In most cases, a healthcare provider will be able to diagnose epidermoid cysts with a physical examination. If the cyst is unusual in presentation, the doctor may order other tests. Rarely, a doctor will order for a biopsy of the tissue sample to test for cancerous cells.

Treatment Of Epidermoid Cysts

If the cyst is painless and does not bother you, it is best to ignore it and not opt for any type of medical intervention. If you do opt for treatment, possible procedures include:

- **Injection:** Medication is injected into the cyst to reduce inflammation and swelling.
- **Incision and drainage:** The doctor cuts the wall of the cyst and drains the contents by squeezing it gently. This treatment is easily done but there is a chance of recurrence.
- **Minor surgery:** Removing a cyst surgically may involve one of three methods:
  - **Conventional wide excision:** The doctor makes a long incision in the skin and removes the entire cysts without draining it. This method ensures that the cyst will not recur, but will likely leave a scar.
  - **Minimal excision:** The doctor makes a small incision, removes the cyst's contents, then removes the walls of the cyst. Scarring is minimal, but the chance of recurrence is higher.
  - **Laser with punch biopsy excision:** The doctor uses a laser to make hole in the surface of the cyst, then drains the contents. After a month, the walls of the cyst are removed.

Complications Of Epidermoid Cysts

The following complications can sometime occur with epidermoid cysts:

- **Inflammation:** Epidermoid cysts tend to become tender and swollen even without infection. Surgical removal will be recommended only after inflammation has subsided.

- **Rupture:** Cyst walls can sometimes break, leading to an infection that and will require prompt medical attention

- **Infection:** Cysts could become infected and cause pain

- **Cancer:** Very rarely, epidermoid cysts can lead to skin cancer

Pilonidal Cysts

A pilonidal cyst is an abnormal pocket of skin that contains hair and skin debris (the term pilonidal means "nest of hair"). This type of cyst usually occurs on the tailbone in or near the cleft of the buttocks. Pilonidal cysts form when hair punctures the skin and becomes embedded. If the cyst becomes infected, the resulting abscess is usually very painful. Pilonidal cysts are common in young men and in people who are obese or who tend to sit for extended periods time, such as truck drivers.

Causes Of Pilonidal Cysts

Doctors believe that pilonidal cysts occur when hairs are forced back into the skin. This can happen when you wear tight clothing, your skin rubs against itself repeatedly, while biking, and long periods of sitting. The skin creates a cyst around the hair, which it considers a foreign substance.

Symptoms Of Pilonidal Cysts

A pilonidal cyst that is infected becomes a swollen mass of tissue that is painful, red, and can have foul-smelling pus and blood drain from it.

Diagnosis Of Pilonidal Cysts

Pilonidal cysts are diagnosed by healthcare professionals with a physical examination. You will be asked questions regarding when and how symptoms began.

Treatment Of Pilonidal Cysts

A healthcare provider will numb the area with an injection, make an incision and drain the fluid inside the cyst. This is commonly done in an outpatient setting. If the cyst recurs, then it will have to be removed surgically. Once the cyst is surgically removed, the doctor may leave the wound open. The surgical site is dressed and allowed to heal on its own. The healing time in such cases is long, but the risk that the cyst comes back is minimal. The doctor in some cases may decide to suture the surgical site (close it using surgical stiches). The healing time in this case is shorter but the risk of recurrence is greater. It is very important to take good care of the wound after surgery. You will have to remove hair from the area that could possibly enter the wound.

Complications Of Pilonidal Cysts

Chronically infected pilonidal cysts have a slight risk of developing a type of skin cancer called squamous cell carcinoma.

Lipoma

A lipoma is a slow-growing fibrous capsule of fat cells found below the skin and above the muscle layer. Lipomas feel doughy, move easily when you apply pressure, and are not tendor or painful. Noncancerous lipomas can be found anywhere in the body but they commonly occur in the chest, neck, armpits, upper arms, and thighs. Lipomas are common, and 1 in 100 people develop this type of cyst. Lipomas generally do not need any sort of medical intervention.

Causes Of Lipomas

The exact cause of lipomas is unknown, but researchers believe there is a genetic factor since lipomas tend to run in families. Lipomas are not connected to being overweight.

Symptoms Of Lipomas

Lipomas can occur anywhere in the body. They have the following features.

- They are small in size and doughy to touch

- It moves and has a soft, rubber-like consistency

- It doesn't change in size or otherwise grows slowly

- It is usually painless but could become painful if it impinges on adjacent nerves or blood vessels

Diagnosis Of Lipomas

A doctor confirms a lipoma by carrying out a physical examination. In very rare instances, a doctor will order further tests if he or she suspects that the mass is not a lipoma but a cancerous growth called a liposarcoma. In the case of liposarcoma, the mass will grow rapidly, will not move, and will cause pain.

Treatment Of Lipomas

No treatment is required for lipoma because it does not cause any pain or other problems. If it hurts or is bothersome, or as a cosmetic purpose, a doctor may decide to surgically remove it. To do so, they will make a small incision and remove the entire lipoma. Generally done using local anaesthetic, the procedure may need to be done under general anaesthetic if the lipoma is not easily accessible. A possible side effect of surgical removal is scarring at the site of incision. Doctors may also use liposuction to remove the mass. Liposuction utilizes a needle and large syringe to remove fatty tissue from under the skin.

References

1. "Cysts (Overview)," Harvard University, October 2012.

2. Delgago, Amanda. "What's Causing This Cyst?" Healthline Media, n.d.

3. "Epidermoid Cysts," Mayo Foundation for Medical Education and Research (MFMER), August 2, 2017.

4. Sullivan, Debra. "What's Causing This Sebaceous Cyst?" Healthline Media, June 14, 2016.

5. Jaliman, Debra, MD. "What Is A Pilonidal Cyst?" WebMD, LLC, October 24, 2016.

6. "Pilonidal Cyst," Mayo Foundation for Medical Education and Research (MFMER), September 5, 2015.

7. "Lipoma," Mayo Foundation for Medical Education and Research (MFMER), January 22, 2015.

8. "Lipoma—Topic Overview," WebMD, LLC, n.d.

Chapter 26

Eczema (Atopic Dermatitis)

What Is Atopic Dermatitis?

Atopic dermatitis is a chronic (long-lasting) disease that affects the skin. It is not contagious; it cannot be passed from one person to another. The word "dermatitis" means inflammation of the skin. "Atopic" refers to a group of diseases in which there is often an inherited tendency to develop other allergic conditions, such as asthma and hay fever. In atopic dermatitis, the skin becomes extremely itchy. Scratching leads to redness, swelling, cracking, "weeping" clear fluid, and finally, crusting and scaling. In most cases, there are periods of time when the disease is worse (called exacerbations or flares) followed by periods when the skin improves or clears up entirely (called remissions). As some children with atopic dermatitis grow older, their skin disease improves or disappears altogether, although their skin often remains dry and easily irritated. In others, atopic dermatitis continues to be a significant problem in adulthood.

Atopic dermatitis is often referred to as "eczema," which is a general term for the several types of inflammation of the skin. Atopic dermatitis is the most common of the many types of eczema. Several have very similar symptoms.

Who Has Atopic Dermatitis?

Atopic dermatitis is very common. It occurs equally in males and females and affects an estimated 30 percent of people in the United States. Although atopic dermatitis may occur at any age, it most often begins in infancy and childhood. Onset after age 30 is less common and

About This Chapter: This chapter includes text excerpted from "Atopic Dermatitis," National Institute of Arthritis and Musculoskeletal and Skin Diseases (NIAMS), July 2016.

is often caused by exposure of the skin to harsh or wet conditions. People who live in cities and in dry climates appear more likely to develop this condition.

Causes Of Atopic Dermatitis

The cause of atopic dermatitis is not known, but the disease seems to result from a combination of genetic (hereditary) and environmental factors.

Children are more likely to develop this disorder if a parent has had it or another atopic disease like asthma or hay fever. If both parents have an atopic disease, the likelihood increases. Although some people outgrow skin symptoms, many children with atopic dermatitis go on to develop hay fever or asthma. Environmental factors can bring on symptoms of atopic dermatitis at any time in affected individuals.

Atopic dermatitis is also associated with malfunction of the body's immune system: the system that recognizes and helps fight bacteria and viruses that invade the body. The immune system can become misguided and create inflammation in the skin, even in the absence of a major infection. This can be viewed as a form of autoimmunity, where a body reacts against its own tissues.

In the past, doctors thought that atopic dermatitis was caused by an emotional disorder. We now know that emotional factors, such as stress, can make the condition worse, but they do not cause the disease.

Symptoms Of Atopic Dermatitis

Symptoms (signs) vary from person to person. The most common symptoms are dry, itchy skin and rashes on the face, inside the elbows and behind the knees, and on the hands and feet. Itching is the most important symptom of atopic dermatitis. Scratching and rubbing in response to itching irritates the skin, increases inflammation, and actually increases itchiness. Itching is a particular problem during sleep when conscious control of scratching is lost.

The appearance of the skin that is affected by atopic dermatitis depends on the amount of scratching and the presence of secondary skin infections. The skin may be red and scaly or thick and leathery, contain small raised bumps, or leak fluid and become crusty and infected. The sidebox below lists common skin features of the disease. These features can also be found in people who do not have atopic dermatitis or who have other types of skin disorders.

Atopic dermatitis may also affect the skin around the eyes, the eyelids, and the eyebrows and lashes. Scratching and rubbing the eye area can cause the skin to redden and swell. Some

Skin Features Associated With Atopic Dermatitis

- **Atopic pleat (Dennie-Morgan fold)**—an extra fold of skin that develops under the eye
- **Cheilitis**—inflammation of the skin on and around the lips
- **Hyperlinear palms**—increased number of skin creases on the palms
- **Hyperpigmented eyelids**—eyelids that have become darker in color from inflammation or hay fever
- **Ichthyosis**—dry, rectangular scales on the skin
- **Keratosis pilaris**—small, rough bumps, generally on the face, upper arms, and thighs
- **Lichenification**—thick, leathery skin resulting from constant scratching and rubbing
- **Papules**—small raised bumps that may open when scratched and become crusty and infected
- **Urticaria**—hives (red, raised bumps) that may occur after exposure to an allergen, at the beginning of flares, or after exercise or a hot bath.

people with atopic dermatitis develop an extra fold of skin under their eyes. Patchy loss of eyebrows and eyelashes may also result from scratching or rubbing.

Researchers have noted differences in the skin of people with atopic dermatitis that may contribute to the symptoms of the disease. The outer layer of skin, called the epidermis, is divided into two parts: an inner part containing moist, living cells, and an outer part, known as the horny layer or stratum corneum, containing dry, flattened, dead cells. Under normal conditions the stratum corneum acts as a barrier, keeping the rest of the skin from drying out and protecting other layers of skin from damage caused by irritants and infections. When this barrier is damaged, irritants act more intensely on the skin.

The skin of a person with atopic dermatitis loses moisture from the epidermal layer, allowing the skin to become very dry and reducing its protective abilities. Thus, when combined with the abnormal skin immune system, the person's skin is more likely to become infected by bacteria or viruses.

Stages Of Atopic Dermatitis

When atopic dermatitis occurs during infancy and childhood, it affects each child differently in terms of both onset and severity of symptoms. In infants, atopic dermatitis typically begins around 6 to 12 weeks of age. It may first appear around the cheeks and chin as a patchy facial rash, which can progress to red, scaling, oozing skin. The skin may become infected.

Once the infant becomes more mobile and begins crawling, exposed areas, such as the inner and outer parts of the arms and legs, may also be affected. An infant with atopic dermatitis may be restless and irritable because of the itching and discomfort of the disease.

In childhood, the rash tends to occur behind the knees and inside the elbows; on the sides of the neck; around the mouth; and on the wrists, ankles, and hands. Often, the rash begins with papules that become hard and scaly when scratched. The skin around the lips may be inflamed, and constant licking of the area may lead to small, painful cracks in the skin around the mouth.

In some children, the disease goes into remission for a long time, only to come back at the onset of puberty when hormones, stress, and the use of irritating skin care products or cosmetics may cause the disease to flare.

Although a number of people who developed atopic dermatitis as children also experience symptoms as adults, it is also possible for the disease to show up first in adulthood. The pattern in adults is similar to that seen in children; that is, the disease may be widespread or limited to only a few parts of the body.

Diagnosing Atopic Dermatitis

Each person with atopic dermatitis experiences a unique combination of symptoms, which may vary in severity over time. The doctor will base a diagnosis on the symptoms the patient experiences and may need to see the patient several times to make an accurate diagnosis and to rule out other diseases and conditions that might cause skin irritation. In some cases, the family doctor or pediatrician may refer the patient to a dermatologist (doctor specializing in skin disorders) or allergist (allergy specialist) for further evaluation.

A medical history may help the doctor better understand the nature of a patient's symptoms, when they occur, and their possible causes. The doctor may ask about family history of allergic disease; whether the patient also has diseases such as hay fever or asthma; and about exposure to irritants, sleep disturbances, any foods that seem to be related to skin flares, previous treatments for skin-related symptoms, and use of steroids or other medications.

Currently, there is no single test to diagnose atopic dermatitis. However, there are some tests that can give the doctor an indication of allergic sensitivity.

Pricking the skin with a needle that contains a small amount of a suspected allergen may be helpful in identifying factors that trigger flares of atopic dermatitis. Negative results on skin tests may help rule out the possibility that certain substances cause skin inflammation. Positive skin prick test results are difficult to interpret in people with atopic dermatitis because the skin is very sensitive to many substances, and there can be many positive test sites that are not meaningful to a person's disease at the time. Positive results simply indicate that the individual has immunoglobulin E or IgE (allergic) antibodies to the substance tested. IgE controls the immune system's allergic response and is often high in atopic dermatitis.

Common Irritants
- Wool or synthetic fibers
- Soaps and detergents
- Some perfumes and cosmetics
- Substances such as chlorine, mineral oil, or solvents
- Dust or sand
- Cigarette smoke

Treatment Of Atopic Dermatitis

The two main goals in treating atopic dermatitis are healing the skin and preventing flares. It is important for the patient and family members to note any changes in the skin's condition in response to treatment, and to be persistent in identifying the treatment that seems to work best.

Medications: A variety of medications are used to treat atopic dermatitis.

Corticosteroid creams and ointments have been used for many years to treat atopic dermatitis and other autoimmune diseases affecting the skin.

When topical corticosteroids are not effective, the doctor may prescribe a systemic corticosteroid, which is taken by mouth or injected instead of being applied directly to the skin. Typically, these medications are used only in resistant cases and only given for short periods of time.

Certain antihistamines that cause drowsiness can reduce nighttime scratching and allow more restful sleep when taken at bedtime. This effect can be particularly helpful for patients whose nighttime scratching makes the disease worse.

Topical calcineurin inhibitors decrease inflammation in the skin and help prevent flares. Barrier repair moisturizers reduce water loss and work to rebuild the skin.

Phototherapy: Use of ultraviolet A or B light waves, alone or combined, can be an effective treatment for mild to moderate dermatitis. If the doctor thinks that phototherapy may be useful to treat the symptoms of atopic dermatitis, he or she will use the minimum exposure necessary and monitor the skin carefully.

Treating Atopic Dermatitis In Infants And Children

- Give lukewarm baths.
- Apply moisturizer immediately following the bath.
- Keep child's fingernails filed short.
- Select soft cotton fabrics when choosing clothing.
- Consider using sedating antihistamines to promote sleep and reduce scratching at night.
- Keep the child cool; avoid situations where overheating occurs.
- Learn to recognize skin infections and seek treatment promptly.
- Attempt to distract the child with activities to keep him or her from scratching.
- Identify and remove irritants and allergens.

Skin care: Healing the skin and keeping it healthy are important to prevent further damage and enhance quality of life. Developing and sticking with a daily skin care routine is critical to preventing flares.

A lukewarm bath helps to cleanse and moisturize the skin without drying it excessively. Because soaps can be drying to the skin, the doctor may recommend use of a mild bar soap or nonsoap cleanser. Bath oils are not usually helpful.

After bathing, a person should air-dry the skin, or pat it dry gently (avoiding rubbing or brisk drying), and then apply a moisturizer to seal in the water that has been absorbed into the skin during bathing. A moisturizer increases the rate of healing and establishes a barrier against further drying and irritation. Lotions that have a high water or alcohol content evaporate more quickly, and alcohol may cause stinging. Creams and ointments work better at healing the skin.

Protection from allergen exposure: The doctor may suggest reducing exposure to a suspected allergen. For example, the presence of the house dust mite can be limited by encasing mattresses and pillows in special dustproof covers, frequently washing bedding in hot water, and removing carpeting. However, there is no way to completely rid the environment of airborne allergens.

Changing the diet may not always relieve symptoms of atopic dermatitis. A change may be helpful, however, when the medical history, laboratory studies, and specific symptoms strongly suggest a food allergy. It is up to the patient and his or her family and physician to decide whether the dietary restrictions are appropriate. Unless properly monitored by a physician or dietitian, diets with many restrictions can contribute to serious nutritional problems, especially in children.

Stress Management: Stress management and relaxation techniques may help decrease the likelihood of flares. Developing a network of support that includes family, friends, health professionals, and support groups or organizations can be beneficial.

Atopic Dermatitis And Vaccination Against Smallpox

Although scientists are working to develop safer vaccines, individuals diagnosed with atopic dermatitis (or eczema) should not receive the current smallpox vaccine. According to the Centers for Disease Control and Prevention (CDC), a U.S. Government organization, individuals who have ever been diagnosed with atopic dermatitis, even if the condition is mild or not presently active, are more likely to develop a serious complication if they are exposed to the virus from the smallpox vaccine.

During a smallpox outbreak, these vaccination recommendations may change. People with atopic dermatitis who have been exposed to smallpox should consult their doctor about vaccination. They should also find out what precautions to take if they have close contact with someone who has recently received the vaccine.

Chapter 27

Epidermolysis Bullosa

What Is Epidermolysis Bullosa (EB)?

Epidermolysis bullosa (EB) is a group of blistering skin conditions. The skin is so fragile in people with epidermolysis bullosa that even minor rubbing may cause blistering. At times, the person with epidermolysis bullosa may not be aware of rubbing or injuring the skin even though blisters develop. In severe epidermolysis bullosa, blisters are not confined to the outer skin. They may develop inside the body, in such places as the linings of the mouth, esophagus, stomach, intestines, upper airway, bladder, and genitals.

The skin has an outer layer called the epidermis and an underlying layer called the dermis. The place where the two layers meet is called the basement membrane zone. The main forms of epidermolysis bullosa are epidermolysis bullosa simplex (EBS), junctional epidermolysis bullosa (JEB), and dystrophic epidermolysis bullosa (DEB). Epidermolysis bullosa simplex occurs in the outer layer of skin; junctional epidermolysis bullosa and dystrophic epidermolysis bullosa occur in the basement membrane zone. These major types of epidermolysis bullosa, which will be described throughout this chapter, also have many subtypes.

Who Gets Epidermolysis Bullosa?

Epidermolysis bullosa occurs in all racial and ethnic groups and affects males and females equally. The disease is not always evident at birth. Milder cases of epidermolysis bullosa may become apparent when a child crawls, walks, or runs, or when a young adult engages in vigorous physical activity.

About This Chapter: This chapter includes text excerpted from "Epidermolysis Bullosa—Questions And Answers About Epidermolysis Bullosa," National Institute of Arthritis and Musculoskeletal and Skin Diseases (NIAMS), November 2016.

What Causes Epidermolysis Bullosa?

Most people with epidermolysis bullosa have inherited the condition through faulty genes they receive from one or both parents. Genes are located in the body's cells and determine inherited traits passed from parent to child. They also govern every body function, such as the formation of proteins in the skin. Several genes are known to underlie the different forms of epidermolysis bullosa. Genes are located on chromosomes, which are structures in each cell's nucleus.

In an autosomal dominant form of epidermolysis bullosa, the disease gene is inherited from only one parent who has the disease, and there is a 50 percent chance (1 in 2) with each pregnancy that a baby will have epidermolysis bullosa. In the autosomal recessive form, the disease gene is inherited from both parents.

Neither parent has to show signs of the disease; they simply need to "carry" the gene, and there is a 25 percent chance (1 in 4) with each pregnancy that a baby will have epidermolysis bullosa. Epidermolysis bullosa can also be acquired through a mutation (abnormal change) in a gene that occurred during the formation of the egg or sperm reproductive cell in a parent. Neither the sex of the child nor the order of birth determines which child or how many children will develop epidermolysis bullosa in a family that has the faulty gene.

Although epidermolysis bullosa simplex can occur when there is no evidence of the disease in the parents, it is usually inherited as an autosomal dominant disease. In epidermolysis bullosa simplex, the faulty genes are those that provide instructions for producing keratin, a fibrous protein in the top layer of skin. As a result, the skin splits in the epidermis, producing a blister.

In junctional epidermolysis bullosa, there is a defect in the genes inherited from both parents (autosomal recessive) that normally promote the formation of anchoring filaments (thread-like fibers) or hemidesmosomes (complex structures composed of many proteins). These structures anchor the epidermis to the underlying basement membrane. The defect leads to tissue separation and blistering in the upper part of the basement membrane.

There are both dominant and recessive forms of dystrophic epidermolysis bullosa. In this condition, the filaments that anchor the epidermis to the underlying dermis are either absent or do not function. This is caused by defects in the gene for type VII collagen, a fibrous protein that is the main component of the anchoring filaments.

Epidermolysis bullosa acquisita (EBA) is a rare autoimmune disorder in which the body attacks its own anchoring fibrils with antibodies, the special proteins that help fight and destroy foreign substances that invade the body. In a few cases, it has occurred following drug therapy for another condition; in most cases, the cause is unknown.

How Is Epidermolysis Bullosa Diagnosed?

Dermatologists can identify where the skin is separating to form blisters and what kind of epidermolysis bullosa a person has by doing a skin biopsy (taking a small sample of skin that is examined under a microscope). One diagnostic test involves use of a microscope and reflected light to see if proteins needed for forming connecting fibrils, filaments, or hemidesmosomes are missing or reduced in number. Another test involves use of a high-power electron microscope, which can greatly magnify tissue images, to identify structural defects in the skin.

Diagnostic techniques make it possible to identify defective genes in epidermolysis bullosa patients and their family members. Prenatal diagnosis can now be accomplished by amniocentesis (removing and examining a small amount of amniotic fluid surrounding the fetus in the womb of a pregnant woman) or sampling the chorionic villus (part of the outer membrane surrounding the fetus) as early as the 10th week of pregnancy.

What Are The Symptoms Of Epidermolysis Bullosa?

The major sign of all forms of epidermolysis bullosa is fragile skin that blisters, which can lead to serious complications. For example, blistering areas may become infected, and blisters in the mouth or parts of the gastrointestinal tract may interfere with proper nutrition.

Following is a summary of some of the characteristic signs of various forms of epidermolysis bullosa.

Epidermolysis Bullosa Simplex

A generalized form of epidermolysis bullosa simplex usually begins with blistering that is evident at birth or shortly afterward. In a localized, mild form called Weber-Cockayne, blisters rarely extend beyond the feet and hands. In some subtypes of epidermolysis bullosa simplex, the blisters occur over widespread areas of the body. Other signs may include thickened skin on the palms of the hands and soles of the feet; rough, thickened, or absent fingernails or toenails; and blistering of the soft tissues inside the mouth. Less common signs include growth retardation; blisters in the esophagus; anemia (a reduction in the red blood cells that carry oxygen to all parts of the body); scarring of the skin; and milia, which are small white skin cysts.

Junctional Epidermolysis Bullosa

This disease is usually severe. In the most serious forms, large, ulcerated blisters on the face, trunk, and legs can be life-threatening because of complicated infections and loss of body fluid that leads to severe dehydration. Survival is also threatened by blisters that affect the esophagus, upper airway, stomach, intestines, and urogenital system. Other signs found in both severe and mild forms of junctional epidermolysis bullosa include rough and thickened or absent fingernails and toenails; a thin appearance to the skin (called atrophic scarring); blisters on the scalp or loss of hair with scarring (scarring alopecia); malnutrition and anemia; growth retardation; involvement of soft tissue inside the mouth and nose; and poorly formed tooth enamel.

Dystrophic Epidermolysis Bullosa

The dominant and recessive inherited forms of dystrophic epidermolysis bullosa have slightly different symptoms. In some dominant and mild recessive forms, blisters may appear only on the hands, feet, elbows, and knees; nails usually are shaped differently; milia may appear on the skin of the trunk and limbs; and there may be involvement of the soft tissues, especially the esophagus. The more severe recessive form is characterized by blisters over large body surfaces, loss of nails or rough or thick nails, atrophic scarring, milia, itching, anemia, and growth retardation. Severe forms of recessive dystrophic epidermolysis bullosa also may lead to severe eye inflammation with erosion of the cornea (clear covering over the front of the eye), early loss of teeth because of tooth decay, and blistering and scarring inside the mouth and gastrointestinal tract. In most people with this form of epidermolysis bullosa, some or all the fingers or toes may fuse (pseudosyndactyly). Also, individuals with recessive dystrophic epidermolysis bullosa have a high risk of developing a form of skin cancer called squamous cell carcinoma. It primarily occurs on the hands and feet. The cancer may begin as early as the teenage years. It tends to grow and spread faster in people with epidermolysis bullosa than in those without the disease.

How Is Epidermolysis Bullosa Treated?

People with mild forms of epidermolysis bullosa may not require extensive treatment. However, they should attempt to keep blisters from forming and prevent infection when blisters occur. Individuals with moderate and severe forms may have many complications and require psychological support along with attention to the care and protection of the skin and soft tissues. Patients, parents, or other care providers should not feel that they must tackle all the complicated aspects of epidermolysis bullosa care alone. There are doctors, nurses, social workers, clergy members, psychologists, dietitians, and patient and parent support groups that can assist with care and provide information and emotional support.

Preventing Blisters

In many forms of epidermolysis bullosa, blisters will form with the slightest pressure or friction. This may make parents hesitant to pick up and cuddle young babies. However, a baby needs to feel a gentle human touch and affection. Parents can learn the best ways to handle babies to minimize the chances of blisters.

A number of things can be done to protect the skin from injury. These include:

- Avoiding overheating by keeping rooms at an even temperature.
- Applying lubricants to the skin to reduce friction and keep the skin moist.
- Using simple, soft clothing that requires minimal handling when dressing a child.
- Using sheepskin on car seats and other hard surfaces.
- Wearing mittens at bedtime to help prevent scratching.

Caring For Blistered Skin

When blisters appear, the objectives of care are to reduce pain or discomfort, prevent excessive loss of body fluid, promote healing, and prevent infection.

The doctor may prescribe a mild analgesic to prevent discomfort during changes of dressings (bandages). Dressings that are sticking to the skin may be removed by soaking them off in warm water. Although daily cleansing may include a bath with mild soaps, it may be more comfortable to bathe in stages where small areas are cleaned at a time.

Blisters can become quite large and create a large wound when they break. Therefore, a medical professional will likely provide instructions on how to safely break a blister in its early stages while still leaving the top skin intact to cover the underlying reddened area. After opening and draining, the doctor may suggest that an antibiotic ointment be applied to the area of the blister before covering it with a sterile, nonsticking bandage. To prevent irritation of the skin from tape, a bandage can be secured with a strip of gauze that is tied around it. In milder cases of epidermolysis bullosa or where areas are difficult to keep covered, the doctor may recommend leaving a punctured blister open to the air.

A moderately moist environment promotes healing, but heavy drainage from blister areas may further irritate the skin, and an absorbent or foam dressing may be needed. There are also contact layer dressings where a mesh layer through which drainage can pass is placed on the wound and is topped by an outer absorbent layer. The doctor or other healthcare professional may recommend gauze or bandages that are soaked with petroleum jelly, glycerin, or lubricating substances, or may suggest more extensive wound care bandages or products.

Treating Infection

The chances of skin infection can be reduced by good nutrition, which builds the body's defenses and promotes healing, and by careful skin care with clean hands and use of sterile materials. For added protection, the doctor may recommend antibiotic ointments and soaks.

Even in the presence of good care, it is possible for infection to develop. Signs of infection are redness and heat around an open area of skin, pus or a yellow drainage, excessive crusting on the wound surface, a red line or streak under the skin that spreads away from the blistered area, a wound that does not heal, and/or fever or chills. The doctor may prescribe a specific soaking solution, an antibiotic ointment, or an oral antibiotic to reduce the growth of bacteria. Wounds that are not healing may be treated by a special wound covering or biologically developed skin.

Treating Nutritional Problems

Blisters that form in the mouth and esophagus in some people with epidermolysis bullosa are likely to cause difficulty in chewing and swallowing food and drinks. If breast or bottle feeding results in blisters, infants may be fed using a preemie nipple (a soft nipple with large holes), a cleft palate nipple, an eyedropper, or a syringe. When the baby is old enough to take in food, adding extra liquid to pureed (finely mashed) food makes it easier to swallow. Soups, milk drinks, mashed potatoes, custards, and puddings can be given to young children. However, food should never be served too hot.

Dietitians are important members of the healthcare team that assists people with epidermolysis bullosa. They can work with family members and older patients to find recipes and prepare food that is nutritious and easy to consume. For example, they can identify high-caloric and protein-fortified foods and beverages that help replace protein lost in the fluid from draining blisters. They can suggest vitamin and mineral nutritional supplements that may be needed, and show how to mix these into the food and drinks of young children. Dietitians can also recommend adjustments in the diet to prevent gastrointestinal problems, such as constipation, diarrhea, or painful elimination.

Surgical Treatment

Surgical treatment may be necessary in some forms of epidermolysis bullosa. Individuals with the severe forms of autosomal recessive dystrophic epidermolysis bullosa whose esophagus has been narrowed by scarring may require dilation of their esophagus for food to travel from the mouth to the stomach. Other individuals who are not getting proper nutrition may need a feeding tube that permits delivery of food directly to the stomach. Also, patients whose fingers or toes are fused together may require surgery to release them.

Chapter 28

Hyperhidrosis (Excessive Sweating)

What Is Hyperhidrosis?

Hyperhidrosis is medical term for excessive sweating that goes beyond a normal response to increased physical activity or a rise in air temperature. Individuals who suffer from the condition may sweat so much that they soak through their clothes or experience sweat dripping from their hands. In some cases, hyperhidrosis affects the whole body, while in others, a person may only experience excessive sweating in specific areas such as the armpits, palms, soles of the feet, groin, chest, or face. If specific areas of the body are involved, then both sides of the body are equally affected. For instance, both right and left palms or both armpits are affected.

When Is Sweating Considered Excessive?

Sweating that regularly interferes with daily activities is considered excessive sweating.

For example:

- You regularly avoid situations that require physical contact, such as shaking hands, because it makes you self-conscious.

- In school or work place, excessive sweating makes it difficult for you to handle instruments and tools, hold onto a steering wheel, or write with a pen or pencil.

- You avoid activities like exercising or dancing because it makes sweating worse.

"Hyperhidrosis (Excessive Sweating)," © 2018 Omnigraphics. Reviewed August 2017.

- Coping with excess sweat takes up a lot of your time. For example, you have to frequently shower or change clothes.

- You have become socially withdrawn and self-conscious because of this condition.

Who Does Hyperhidrosis Affect?

Hyperhidrosis affects people of all ages. Researchers estimate that 2 to 3 percent of the world population has suffered from hyperhidrosis at some point in their lives. Most of those who suffer from hyperhidrosis are unaware of treatment options, and therefore, half of all cases are never diagnosed or treated.

What Are The Symptoms Of Hyperhidrosis?

Most people sweat when it is hot, during physical exertion, or when they are nervous, anxious, or under stress. People with hyperhidrosis, however, produce far more sweat under these conditions and also tend to sweat for no apparent reason. People who overproduce sweat in specific areas tend to experience at least one episode of excessive sweating in a week during waking hours.

When Should You Call A Doctor?

If excessive sweating regularly interferes with your day-to-day life, you and your parents should contact your doctor about possible solutions. People with hyperhidrosis tend to believe that nothing can be done about their condition. However, treatment options do exist.

You should also call your doctor immediately if excessive sweating is accompanied by a high fever, chills, nausea, lightheadedness, or chest pain since this may signal that you have a more serious condition, such as a bacterial or viral infection.

How Do Doctors Diagnose Hyperhidrosis?

A doctor will perform a physical examination first and follow up with a range of other tests for diagnosis.

- **Starch-iodine test:** Doctors apply an iodine solution to an area of the body, such as palms or underarms, and then sprinkle starch on it. If the combination turns dark blue, excess production of sweat is occurring in the area.

- **Paper test:** Doctors place a special paper on the affected area to absorb sweat. The paper is later weighed to determine how much sweat was produced.

- **Laboratory tests:** Doctors will order regular tests to determine if an undiagnosed condition or illness is the underlying cause. These include thyroid, blood glucose, uric acid, and urine tests.

What Causes Hyperhidrosis?

Everyone's skin contains millions of sweat glands. They help regulate the temperature of our bodies by releasing sweat that then evaporates from the surface of the skin, cooling the body down. The autonomic nervous system, the part of the nervous system that automatically controls our bodily functions, regulates this process.

Researchers believe that hyperhidrosis stems from the autonomic nervous system over-stimulating a specific type of sweat gland, known as eccrine glands, in response to stimulation such as rise in temperature, stress, or physical activity. The nervous system may even trigger perspiration when not warranted.

Depending on the root cause of that overstimulation, doctors classify hyperhidrosis is into one of two categories:

- Primary hyperhidrosis—No underlying condition or disease can be found. Excessive sweating limited to particular body parts is normally associated with primary hyperhidrosis. Doctors also suspect that primary hyperhidrosis could be inherited.

- Secondary hyperhidrosis—Excessive sweating can be traced to an underlying condition, such as:

- Certain types of cancer and nervous system disorders:

  - Diabetes

  - Low blood sugar

  - Heart attack

  - Infectious diseases

  - Medications

Secondary hyperhidrosis is usually characterized by excessive sweating all over.

How Do Doctors Treat Hyperhidrosis?

The goal of treatment is to control excessive sweating. If an underlying condition exists, then doctors will focus on treating that condition. If, however, no such condition exists, then treatment focuses on decreasing the severity of the problem. While treatment can be successful, there is a chance that symptoms may reoccur and you may have to undergo ongoing therapy to control symptoms.

The following treatments are used alone or in combination for hyperhidrosis.

Medications

Antiperspirants: If regular antiperspirants are not working, the doctor will prescribe medicinal strength antiperspirant with aluminum chloride such as Drysol and Xerac AC. You apply on the skin before going to bed and wash it off in the morning. Aluminum chloride causes mild skin irritation.

Anticholinergics: A doctor could prescribe medications that block nerve signals so as to prevent the nervous system from activating the sweat glands. These drugs, known as anticholinergics, work by acting on a chemical called acetylcholine in the nervous system. Anticholinergics are available in tablet and solution for. Propantheline bromide is an anticholinergic licensed for the treatment of hyperhidrosis. Some anticholinergics, such as oxybutynin and glycopyrronium bromide, are not licensed for use for the treatment of hyperhidrosis, but doctors may prescribe them if they think the patient benefit. Side effects such as dry mouth, blurred vision, and bladder problems.

Antidepressants: Certain medications used for the treatment of depression decrease sweating. In addition, they reduce anxiety in individuals experiencing social problems related to hyperhidrosis.

Botulinum Toxin: Botulinum toxin injections (Botox, Myobloc) used to treat facial wrinkles can be used to treat hyperhidrosis as well. The injections block neural impulses from the brain to the sweat glands, thereby reducing sweating. A doctor will administer several injections under local anesthetic to affected areas of the body. The effects of the toxin last from 6 to 12 months, after which the treatment regimen is repeated. Side effects to the toxin are mostly short lived.

Surgical Procedures

Surgery is the final alternative treatment and only recommended in severe cases when other forms of treatments have failed to address the condition.

Removal of sweat glands: To treat excessive sweating in the armpits, surgeons can remove the sweat glands under local anesthetic by suctioning, cutting, or scraping them out.

Nerve surgery: In this procedure, the surgeon severs the nerves that connect to the sweat glands. This is a very effective form of treatment but not without side effects. In some cases, it results in excessive sweating in other areas of the body. This form of treatment is considered a last resort when all other forms of treatment have failed to provide the needed relief.

Other Procedures

Iontophoresis: This procedure uses an electric current run through water to treat hyperhidrosis. While experts do not completely understand how the treatment works, they believe the current blocks the sweat glands. To treat hands and feet, the patient will stand or immerse their hands in a shallow water bath while the current runs through the water. For armpits, a medical professional will apply a wet pad, which then has a current run through it. The treatment is painless, but it could cause irritation for a short time. Each session lasts for 20 to 30 minutes and initial treatment usually requires two to four sessions in a week. If symptoms begin to improve, treatment continues in intervals of one to four weeks based on severity of the condition.

Emerging Treatment Procedures

New treatment procedures that use ultrasound, microwave, and laser technologies are making an appearance in the treatment of hyperhidrosis.

How To Cope With Hyperhidrosis?

To alleviate the symptoms of hyperhidrosis, you can also take the following steps:

- Bathe daily.

- Use antiperspirant regularly.

- Wear shoes and socks made out of natural materials.

- Wear multiple pairs of shoes and regularly rotate wearing them.

- Change socks frequently.

- Wear sandals when they are an option. Stay barefooted whenever possible.

- Wear fabrics that are suitable for specific activities. Wear material that will allow your skin to breathe and, for strenuous activities, wear material that will wick body moisture away.

- Use relaxation techniques to keep yourself calm and prevent nervousness.

References

1. Ratini, Melinda, DO, MS. "Hyperhidrosis (Excessive Sweating)," WebMD, LLC, August 2016.

2. "Hyperhidrosis," Mayo Foundation for Medical Education and Research (MFMER), August 18, 2015.

3. "Hyperhidrosis," Cleveland Clinic, 2017.

4. "Hyperhidrosis," NHS Choices, June 1, 2015.

Chapter 29

Keloids

A keloid is a type of scar that forms as a result of an abnormal wound-healing mechanism of the skin. Characterized by a benign fibrous outgrowth that extends beyond the original trauma site and invades healthy skin, keloid usually results from deep injuries, such as those associated with surgical incisions, burns, piercings, lacerations, or sometimes, even acne. Keloid scars happen when fibroblasts (connective tissue cells) multiply at an abnormally high rate, which in turn leads to an excessive production of collagen—the main structural protein involved in wound healing.

Keloid scars commonly affect the upper torso, including the neck, arms, chest, back, and earlobes, and they do not fade spontaneously as do normal scars. Along with the body image implications associated with them, keloids can also cause functional deformities. For instance, keloids over a joint can restrict movement and affect a person's quality of life.

Causes

While the exact cause of keloid remains largely unknown, researchers believe it has a genetic component. Further, ethnicity is also an important indicator as seen in the higher incidence of keloid among dark-skinned people. Cases of spontaneous keloid scarring in the absence of any previous injury, although rare, have also been reported.

Symptoms

Keloid scars appear as well-defined, firm, nodular, rubbery lesions that are raised as high as a quarter of an inch from the body surface. They are shiny and may range in appearance from pink to red, or even brown. While a few may be asymptomatic and harmless, others may be associated with symptoms, including stiffness; pain; pruritis (itchiness); and hyperesthesia (increased physical sensitivity).

> Scars usually fade over time but never go away completely. If the way a scar looks bothers you, various treatments might minimize it. These include surgical revision, dermabrasion, laser treatments, injections, chemical peels, and creams.
>
> *(Source: "Scars," MedlinePlus, National Institutes of Health (NIH).)*

Treatment

Although a wide range of therapies—both invasive and noninvasive—have been used to treat keloids, none of the current treatment methods can guarantee a complete cure or prevent recurrence.

Noninvasive Therapy

Pressure Garments Therapy (PGT): A standard treatment for keloid, this involves application of continuous pressure on the scar using a tight-fitting garment for a period of six months to a year, which is generally the time taken between wound closure and scar maturation. The lengthy duration and the discomfort associated with this treatment have restricted its use in clinical practice.

Silicone Gel: A relatively recent treatment for keloid scars, this is a self-drying topical application that works by reducing collagen synthesis, keeping the skin hydrated, and regulating growth factors that help to break down the excess collagen in the scar tissue. Silicone gels also protect the scar from bacterial infection and help relieve the itching and discomfort generally associated with keloids.

Corticosteroid therapy: Steroids work by repressing mitosis (cell division) and inflammation. Widely used as a first line treatment for prevention and treatment of keloid scars, they are injected directly into the lesion and are typically combined with other treatments, such as cryotherapy, or surgery for better outcomes.

Invasive Therapy

Surgery: This is the most common type of invasive treatment for scar revision. However, it is seldom used as a stand-alone treatment since the risk of recurrence is significant. Further, the surgical site may produce a larger lesion than the original keloid. To circumvent this, surgery is usually accompanied by other complimentary treatments, such as steroid or radiotherapy. Surgery may involve either a simple removal of the scar tissue followed by primary closure (suturing of the skin edges of the wound); or a wide margin excision of the scar followed by closure using a skin graft taken from another part of the patient's body.

Cryotherapy: A standard treatment protocol for keloids, either as standalone treatment or in combination with corticosteroids, cryotherapy is particularly useful in treating smaller or recently formed lesions. The procedure is based on the application of extremely low temperatures to induce damage, and eventually, necrosis (death) of the abnormal scar tissue. A probe or needle attached to a source of liquid nitrogen is inserted deep into the scar tissue. The needle freezes over and, in turn, freezes the scar tissue from inside. Cryotherapy has been linked to significant reduction in scar volume and alleviation of pain and discomfort associated with keloid.

Prevention

Prevention is as critical as management given the clinical challenges and singular lack of completely effective treatments for keloid scars. Avoiding nonessential cosmetic procedures, such as tattooing or skin piercing is particularly important for people with a history of keloids. Using specialized surgical techniques to treat high-risk individuals is an important part of prevention, as is meticulous postoperative wound care that employs specific measures to minimize scarring, such as pressure garments and silicone products.

References

1. "Keloids," American Academy of Dermatology, n.d.

2. Juckett, Gregory, MD, MPH, Hartman-Adams, Holly, MD. "Management Of Keloids And Hypertrophic Scars," American Academy of Family Physicians (AAFP), August 1, 2009.

3. Hunasgi, Santosh, Koneru, Anila, Vanishree M., Shamala, Ravikumar. "Keloid: A Case Report And Review Of Pathophysiology And Differences Between Keloid And Hypertrophic Scars," National Center for Biotechnology Information (NCBI), n.d.

4. Sukari Halim, Ahmad, Emami, Azadeh, Salahshourifar, Iman, Ponnuraj Kannan, Thirumulu. "Keloid Scarring: Understanding The Genetic Basis, Advances, And Prospects," National Center for Biotechnology Information (NCBI), n.d.

Chapter 30

Lupus

Lupus is an autoimmune disease that triggers inflammation in different tissues of the body. Autoimmune diseases happen when the body's immune system attacks its own tissues. The most common type of lupus is systemic lupus erythematosus (SLE), which affects different parts of the body including internal organs.

Systemic Lupus Erythematosus (SLE)

What Is Systemic Lupus Erythematosus (SLE)?

SLE, a type of lupus, is an autoimmune disease in which the immune system attacks its own tissues. It can affect the joints, skin, brain, lungs, kidneys, and blood vessels, and can cause widespread inflammation and tissue damage in the affected organs. There is no cure for lupus, but medical interventions and lifestyle changes can help control it.

How Serious Is SLE?

The seriousness of SLE can range from mild to life-threatening. The disease should be treated by a doctor or a team of doctors who specialize in care of SLE patients. People with lupus that get proper medical care, preventive care, and education can significantly improve function and quality of life.

What Causes SLE?

The causes of SLE are unknown, but are believed to be linked to environmental, genetic, and hormonal factors.

About This Chapter: This chapter includes text excerpted from "Lupus—Lupus Detailed Fact Sheet," Centers for Disease Control and Prevention (CDC), January 30, 2017.

What Are The Signs And Symptoms?

People with SLE may experience a variety of symptoms that include fatigue, skin rashes, fevers, and pain or swelling in the joints. SLE symptoms may affect women and men differently. Among some adults, having a period of SLE symptoms—called flares—may happen every so often, sometimes even years apart, and go away at other times—called remission. However, other adults may experience SLE flares more frequently throughout their life.

Other symptoms can include sun sensitivity, oral ulcers, arthritis, lung problems, heart problems, kidney problems, seizures, psychosis, and blood cell and immunological abnormalities.

What Are The Complications Of SLE?

SLE can have both short- and long-term effects on a person's life. Early diagnosis and effective treatments can help reduce the damaging effects of SLE and improve the chance to have better function and quality of life. Poor access to care, late diagnosis, less effective treatments, and poor adherence to therapeutic regimens may increase the damaging effects of SLE, causing more complications and an increased risk of death.

SLE can limit a person's physical, mental, and social functioning. These limitations experienced by women and men with SLE can impact their quality of life, especially if they experience fatigue. Fatigue is the most common symptom affecting the quality of life of people with SLE.

Many studies use employment as a measure to determine the quality of life of people with SLE as employment is central to a person's life. Some studies have shown that the longer a person has had SLE, the less likely they are to be a part of the workforce. On average only 46 percent of people with SLE of working age report being employed.

Adherence to treatment regimens is often a problem, especially among young, reproductive age women. Because SLE treatment may require the use of strong immunosuppressive medications that can have serious side effects, female patients must stop taking the medication before and during pregnancy to protect unborn children from harm.

SLE Diagnosis

How Is SLE Diagnosed?

SLE is diagnosed by a healthcare provider using symptom assessments, physical examination, X-rays, and lab tests. SLE may be difficult to diagnose because its signs and symptoms are not specific and can look like signs and symptoms of other diseases. SLE may also be misdiagnosed if only a blood test is used for diagnosis. Because diagnosis can be challenging, it is important to see a doctor specializing in rheumatology for a final diagnosis. Rheumatologists sometimes use specific criteria for diagnosing SLE.

Who Is At Risk For SLE?

SLE can affect people of all ages, including children. However, women of childbearing ages—15 to 44 years—are at greatest risk of developing SLE. Women are affected far more than men (estimates range from 4 to 12 women for every 1 man).

Minority and ethnic groups—blacks/African Americans, Hispanics/Latinos, Asians, and American Indians/Alaska Natives—are affected more than whites.

Does SLE Run In Families?

Most people with SLE do not have family members with the disease; however, some people with SLE do have a family history of the disease. Men and women with an immediate family member with SLE have only a slightly higher risk for the disease.

SLE Treatment

How Is SLE Treated?

A team approach in treating SLE is often needed because of the number of organs that can be involved.

SLE treatment consists primarily of immunosuppressive drugs that inhibit activity of the immune system. Hydroxychloroquine and corticosteroids (e.g., prednisone) are often used to treat SLE. The U.S. Food and Drug Administration (FDA) approved belimumab in 2011, the first new drug for SLE in more than 50 years.

SLE also may occur with other autoimmune conditions that require additional treatments, like Sjogren syndrome, antiphospholipid syndrome, thyroiditis, hemolytic anemia, and idiopathic thrombocytopenia purpura.

SLE Prevalence And Incidence

Prevalence is a measurement of all individuals affected by the disease at a particular time. Incidence is a measurement of the number of new cases of individuals who contract a disease during a particular period of time, often a year.

Recent national estimates of prevalence and incidence are not available. SLE is relatively uncommon and not a reportable disease, so it is relatively expensive to capture all diagnosed cases reliably for epidemiologic studies. There are no recent studies to determine if SLE prevalence or incidence are changing over time.

Mortality

Causes of premature death associated with SLE are mainly active disease, organ failure (e.g., kidneys), infection, or cardiovascular disease from accelerated atherosclerosis. In a large international SLE cohort with average follow-up of over 8 years during a 1958–2001 observation interval, observed deaths were much higher than expected for all causes, and in particular for circulatory disease, infections, renal disease, and some cancers. Those who were female, younger, and had SLE of short duration were at higher risk of SLE-associated mortality.

Using death certificates for U.S. residents, SLE was identified as the underlying cause of death for an average of 1,034 deaths from 2010–2014. SLE was identified as a contributing cause of death (one of multiple causes of death, including underlying cause of death) for an average of 1,803 deaths during that 4-year-period.

Other Types Of Lupus

SLE is the most common and most serious type of lupus. Other types of lupus include the following:

Cutaneous lupus (skin lupus) is lupus that affects the skin in the form of a rash or lesions. This type of lupus can occur on any part of the body, but usually appears where the skin is exposed to sunlight.

Drug-induced lupus is similar to SLE, but occurs as the result of an overreaction to certain medications. Symptoms usually occur 3 to 6 months after starting a medication, and disappear once the medicine is stopped.

Neonatal lupus occurs when an infant passively acquires autoantibodies from a mother with SLE. The skin, liver, and blood problems resolve by 6 months, but the most serious sign—congenital heart block—requires a pacemaker and has a mortality rate of about 20 percent.

Chapter 31

Skin Cancer

What Is Skin Cancer?[1]

The skin is the body's largest organ. It protects against heat, sunlight, injury, and infection. Skin also helps control body temperature and stores water, fat, and vitamin D. The skin has several layers, but the two main layers are the epidermis (upper or outer layer) and the dermis (lower or inner layer). Skin cancer begins in the epidermis, which is made up of three kinds of cells:

- **Squamous cells:** Thin, flat cells that form the top layer of the epidermis.

- **Basal cells:** Round cells under the squamous cells.

- **Melanocytes:** Cells that make melanin and are found in the lower part of the epidermis. Melanin is the pigment that gives skin its natural color. When skin is exposed to the sun, melanocytes make more pigment and cause the skin to darken.

Skin cancer can occur anywhere on the body, but it is most common in skin that is often exposed to sunlight, such as the face, neck, hands, and arms.

There Are Different Types Of Cancer That Start In The Skin

The most common types are basal cell carcinoma and squamous cell carcinoma, which are nonmelanoma skin cancers. Nonmelanoma skin cancers rarely spread to other parts of the body. Melanoma is a much rarer type of skin cancer. It is more likely to invade nearby tissues

About This Chapter: This chapter includes text excerpted from documents published by two public domain sources. Text under headings marked 1 are excerpted from "Skin Cancer Treatment (PDQ®)–Patient Version," National Cancer Institute (NCI), July 12, 2017; Text under the heading marked 2 is excerpted from "Melanoma Treatment (PDQ®)–Patient Version," National Cancer Institute (NCI), June 16, 2017.

and spread to other parts of the body. Actinic keratosis is a skin condition that sometimes becomes squamous cell carcinoma.

Skin Color And Being Exposed To Sunlight Can Increase The Risk Of Nonmelanoma Skin Cancer And Actinic Keratosis

Anything that increases your chance of getting a disease is called a risk factor. Having a risk factor does not mean that you will get cancer; not having risk factors doesn't mean that you will not get cancer. Talk with your doctor if you think you may be at risk.

Risk factors for basal cell carcinoma and squamous cell carcinoma include the following:

- Being exposed to natural sunlight or artificial sunlight (such as from tanning beds) over long periods of time.

- Having a fair complexion, which includes the following:

  - Fair skin that freckles and burns easily, does not tan, or tans poorly.

  - Blue or green or other light-colored eyes.

  - Red or blond hair.

- Having actinic keratosis.

- Past treatment with radiation.

- Having a weakened immune system.

- Having certain changes in the genes that are linked to skin cancer.

- Being exposed to arsenic.

Risk factors for actinic keratosis include the following:

- Being exposed to natural sunlight or artificial sunlight (such as from tanning beds) over long periods of time.

- Having a fair complexion, which includes the following:

  - Fair skin that freckles and burns easily, does not tan, or tans poorly.

  - Blue or green or other light-colored eyes.

  - Red or blond hair.

Although having a fair complexion is a risk factor for skin cancer and actinic keratosis, people of all skin colors can get skin cancer and actinic keratosis.

Nonmelanoma Skin Cancer And Actinic Keratosis Often Appear As A Change In The Skin

Not all changes in the skin are a sign of nonmelanoma skin cancer or actinic keratosis. Check with your doctor if you notice any changes in your skin.

Signs of nonmelanoma skin cancer include the following:

- A sore that does not heal.
- Areas of the skin that are:
  - Raised, smooth, shiny, and look pearly.
  - Firm and look like a scar, and may be white, yellow, or waxy.
  - Raised, and red or reddish-brown.
  - Scaly, bleeding or crusty.

Signs of actinic keratosis include the following:

- A rough, red, pink, or brown, raised, scaly patch on the skin that may be flat or raised.
- Cracking or peeling of the lower lip that is not helped by lip balm or petroleum jelly.

Tests Or Procedures That Examine The Skin Are Used To Detect (Find) And Diagnose Nonmelanoma Skin Cancer And Actinic Keratosis

The following procedures may be used:

- **Skin exam:** A doctor or nurse checks the skin for bumps or spots that look abnormal in color, size, shape, or texture.
- **Skin biopsy:** All or part of the abnormal-looking growth is cut from the skin and viewed under a microscope by a pathologist to check for signs of cancer. There are four main types of skin biopsies:
  - **Shave biopsy:** A sterile razor blade is used to "shave-off" the abnormal-looking growth.
  - **Punch biopsy:** A special instrument called a punch or a trephine is used to remove a circle of tissue from the abnormal-looking growth.
  - **Incisional biopsy:** A scalpel is used to remove part of a growth.
  - **Excisional biopsy:** A scalpel is used to remove the entire growth.

Certain Factors Affect Prognosis (Chance Of Recovery) And Treatment Options

The prognosis (chance of recovery) depends mostly on the stage of the cancer and the type of treatment used to remove the cancer.

Treatment options depend on the following:

- The stage of the cancer (whether it has spread deeper into the skin or to other places in the body).

- The type of cancer.

- The size of the tumor and what part of the body it affects.

- The patient's general health.

Stages Of Skin Cancer[1]

The process used to find out if cancer has spread within the skin or to other parts of the body is called staging. The information gathered from the staging process determines the stage of the disease. It is important to know the stage in order to plan treatment.

The following tests and procedures may be used in the staging process:

- **CT scan (CAT scan):** A procedure that makes a series of detailed pictures of areas inside the body, taken from different angles. The pictures are made by a computer linked to an X-ray machine.

- **MRI (magnetic resonance imaging):** A procedure that uses a magnet, radio waves, and a computer to make a series of detailed pictures of areas inside the body.

- **Lymph node biopsy:** For squamous cell carcinoma, the lymph nodes may be removed and checked to see if cancer has spread to them.

There Are Three Ways That Cancer Spreads In The Body

- Tissue. The cancer spreads from where it began by growing into nearby areas.

- Lymph system. The cancer spreads from where it began by getting into the lymph system. The cancer travels through the lymph vessels to other parts of the body.

- Blood. The cancer spreads from where it began by getting into the blood. The cancer travels through the blood vessels to other parts of the body.

Cancer May Spread From Where It Began To Other Parts Of The Body

When cancer spreads to another part of the body, it is called metastasis. Cancer cells break away from where they began (the primary tumor) and travel through the lymph system or blood.

When cancer spreads to another part of the body, it is called metastasis. Cancer cells break away from where they began (the primary tumor) and travel through the lymph system or blood.

Staging Of Nonmelanoma Skin Cancer Depends On Whether The Tumor Has Certain "High-Risk" Features And If The Tumor Is On The Eyelid

Staging for nonmelanoma skin cancer that is on the eyelid is different from staging for nonmelanoma skin cancer that affects other parts of the body.

The following are high-risk features for nonmelanoma skin cancer that is not on the eyelid:

- The tumor is thicker than 2 millimeters.
- The tumor is described as Clark level IV (has spread into the lower layer of the dermis) or Clark level V (has spread into the layer of fat below the skin).
- The tumor has grown and spread along nerve pathways.
- The tumor began on an ear or on a lip that has hair on it.
- The tumor has cells that look very different from normal cells under a microscope.

The Following Stages Are Used For Nonmelanoma Skin Cancer That Is Not On The Eyelid

Stage 0 (Carcinoma In Situ)

In stage 0, abnormal cells are found in the squamous cell or basal cell layer of the epidermis (topmost layer of the skin). These abnormal cells may become cancer and spread into nearby normal tissue. Stage 0 is also called carcinoma in situ.

Stage I

In stage I, cancer has formed. The tumor is not larger than 2 centimeters at its widest point and may have one high-risk feature.

Stage II

In stage II, the tumor is either:

- larger than 2 centimeters at its widest point; or

- any size and has two or more high-risk features.

Stage III

In stage III:

- The tumor has spread to the jaw, eye socket, or side of the skull. Cancer may have spread to one lymph node on the same side of the body as the tumor. The lymph node is not larger than 3 centimeters.

  or

- Cancer has spread to one lymph node on the same side of the body as the tumor. The lymph node is not larger than 3 centimeters and one of the following is true:

  - the tumor is not larger than 2 centimeters at its widest point and may have one high-risk feature; or

  - the tumor is larger than 2 centimeters at its widest point; or

  - the tumor is any size and has two or more high-risk features.

Stage IV

In stage IV, one of the following is true:

- The tumor is any size and may have spread to the jaw, eye socket, or side of the skull. Cancer has spread to one lymph node on the same side of the body as the tumor and the affected node is larger than 3 centimeters but not larger than 6 centimeters, or cancer has spread to more than one lymph node on one or both sides of the body and the affected nodes are not larger than 6 centimeters; or

- The tumor is any size and may have spread to the jaw, eye socket, skull, spine, or ribs. Cancer has spread to one lymph node that is larger than 6 centimeters; or

- The tumor is any size and has spread to the base of the skull, spine, or ribs. Cancer may have spread to the lymph nodes; or

- Cancer has spread to other parts of the body, such as the lung.

The Following Stages Are Used For Nonmelanoma Skin Cancer On The Eyelid

Stage 0 (Carcinoma In Situ)

In stage 0, abnormal cells are found in the epidermis (topmost layer of the skin). These abnormal cells may become cancer and spread into nearby normal tissue. Stage 0 is also called carcinoma in situ.

Stage I

Stage I is divided into stages IA, IB, and IC.

- Stage IA: The tumor is 5 millimeters or smaller and has not spread to the connective tissue of the eyelid or to the edge of the eyelid where the lashes are.

- Stage IB: The tumor is larger than 5 millimeters but not larger than 10 millimeters or has spread to the connective tissue of the eyelid, or to the edge of the eyelid where the lashes are.

- Stage IC: The tumor is larger than 10 millimeters but not larger than 20 millimeters or has spread through the full thickness of the eyelid.

Stage II

In stage II, one of the following is true:

- The tumor is larger than 20 millimeters.

- The tumor has spread to nearby parts of the eye or eye socket.

- The tumor has spread to spaces around the nerves in the eyelid.

Stage III

Stage III is divided into stages IIIA, IIIB, and IIIC.

- Stage IIIA: To remove all of the tumor, the whole eye and part of the optic nerve must be removed. The bone, muscles, fat, and connective tissue around the eye may also be removed.

- Stage IIIB: The tumor may be anywhere in or near the eye and has spread to nearby lymph nodes.

- Stage IIIC: The tumor has spread to structures around the eye or in the face, or to the brain, and cannot be removed in surgery.

Stage IV

The tumor has spread to distant parts of the body.

Treatment Is Based On The Type Of Nonmelanoma Skin Cancer Or Other Skin Condition Diagnosed

Basal Cell Carcinoma

Basal cell carcinoma is the most common type of skin cancer. It usually occurs on areas of the skin that have been in the sun, most often the nose. Often this cancer appears as a raised bump that looks smooth and pearly. Another type looks like a scar and is flat and firm and may be white, yellow, or waxy. Basal cell carcinoma may spread to tissues around the cancer, but it usually does not spread to other parts of the body.

Squamous Cell Carcinoma

Squamous cell carcinoma occurs on areas of the skin that have been in the sun, such as the ears, lower lip, and the back of the hands. Squamous cell carcinoma may also appear on areas of the skin that have been burned or exposed to chemicals or radiation. Often this cancer appears as a firm red bump. The tumor may feel scaly, bleed, or form a crust. Squamous cell tumors may spread to nearby lymph nodes. Squamous cell carcinoma that has not spread can usually be cured.

Actinic Keratosis

Actinic keratosis is a skin condition that is not cancer, but sometimes changes into squamous cell carcinoma. It usually occurs in areas that have been exposed to the sun, such as the face, the back of the hands, and the lower lip. It looks like rough, red, pink, or brown scaly patches on the skin that may be flat or raised, or the lower lip cracks and peels and is not helped by lip balm or petroleum jelly.

Treatment Option Overview[1]

Different types of treatment are available for patients with nonmelanoma skin cancer and actinic keratosis. Some treatments are standard (the currently used treatment), and some are being tested in clinical trials. A treatment clinical trial is a research study meant to help improve current treatments or obtain information on new treatments for patients with cancer. When clinical trials show that a new treatment is better than the standard treatment, the new treatment may become the standard treatment. Patients may want to think about taking part in a clinical trial. Some clinical trials are open only to patients who have not started treatment.

Six Types Of Standard Treatment Are Used

1. Surgery

    One or more of the following surgical procedures may be used to treat nonmelanoma skin cancer or actinic keratosis:

    *   Mohs micrographic surgery: The tumor is cut from the skin in thin layers. During surgery, the edges of the tumor and each layer of tumor removed are viewed through a microscope to check for cancer cells.

    *   Simple excision: The tumor is cut from the skin along with some of the normal skin around it.

    *   Shave excision: The abnormal area is shaved off the surface of the skin with a small blade.

    *   Electrodesiccation and curettage: The tumor is cut from the skin with a curette (a sharp, spoon-shaped tool). A needle-shaped electrode is then used to treat the area with an electric current that stops the bleeding and destroys cancer cells that remain around the edge of the wound.

    *   Cryosurgery: A treatment that uses an instrument to freeze and destroy abnormal tissue, such as carcinoma in situ.

    *   Laser surgery: A surgical procedure that uses a laser beam (a narrow beam of intense light) as a knife to make bloodless cuts in tissue or to remove a surface lesion such as a tumor.

    *   Dermabrasion: Removal of the top layer of skin using a rotating wheel or small particles to rub away skin cells.

2. Radiation therapy

    Radiation therapy is a cancer treatment that uses high-energy X-rays or other types of radiation to kill cancer cells or keep them from growing. There are two types of radiation therapy:

    *   External radiation therapy uses a machine outside the body to send radiation toward the cancer.

    *   Internal radiation therapy uses a radioactive substance sealed in needles, seeds, wires, or catheters that are placed directly into or near the cancer.

    The way the radiation therapy is given depends on the type of cancer being treated. External radiation therapy is used to treat skin cancer.

3. Chemotherapy

   Chemotherapy is a cancer treatment that uses drugs to stop the growth of cancer cells, either by killing the cells or by stopping them from dividing.

4. Photodynamic therapy

   Photodynamic therapy (PDT) is a cancer treatment that uses a drug and a certain type of laser light to kill cancer cells.

5. Biologic therapy

   Biologic therapy is a treatment that uses the patient's immune system to fight cancer. Substances made by the body or made in a laboratory are used to boost, direct, or restore the body's natural defenses against cancer.

6. Targeted therapy

   Targeted therapy is a type of treatment that uses drugs or other substances to attack cancer cells.

Follow-Up Tests May Be Needed

Some of the tests that were done to diagnose the cancer or to find out the stage of the cancer may be repeated. Some tests will be repeated in order to see how well the treatment is working. Decisions about whether to continue, change, or stop treatment may be based on the results of these tests.

Some of the tests will continue to be done from time to time after treatment has ended. The results of these tests can show if your condition has changed or if the cancer has recurred (come back). These tests are sometimes called follow-up tests or check-ups.

Basal cell carcinoma and squamous cell carcinoma are likely to recur (come back), usually within 5 years, or new tumors may form. Talk to your doctor about how often you should have your skin checked for signs of cancer.

Treatment Options For Nonmelanoma Skin Cancer[1]

Basal Cell Carcinoma

Treatment of basal cell carcinoma may include the following:

• Simple excision

- Mohs micrographic surgery
- Radiation therapy
- Electrodesiccation and curettage
- Cryosurgery
- Photodynamic therapy
- Topical chemotherapy
- Topical biologic therapy with imiquimod
- Laser surgery

Treatment of recurrent basal cell carcinoma is usually Mohs micrographic surgery.

Treatment of basal cell carcinoma that is metastatic or cannot be treated with local therapy may include the following:

- Targeted therapy with a signal transduction inhibitor
- Chemotherapy
- A clinical trial of a new treatment

Squamous Cell Carcinoma

Treatment of squamous cell carcinoma may include the following:

- Simple excision
- Mohs micrographic surgery
- Radiation therapy
- Electrodesiccation and curettage
- Cryosurgery

Treatment of recurrent squamous cell carcinoma may include the following:

- Simple excision
- Mohs micrographic surgery
- Radiation therapy

Treatment of squamous cell carcinoma that is metastatic or cannot be treated with local therapy may include the following:

- Chemotherapy

- Retinoid therapy and biologic therapy with interferon

- A clinical trial of a new treatment

Treatment Options For Melanoma Skin Cancer[2]

Melanoma is a disease in which malignant (cancer) cells form in melanocytes (cells that color the skin)

The skin is the body's largest organ. It protects against heat, sunlight, injury, and infection. Skin also helps control body temperature and stores water, fat, and vitamin D. The skin has several layers, but the two main layers are the epidermis (upper or outer layer) and the dermis (lower or inner layer). Skin cancer begins in the epidermis, which is made up of three kinds of cells:

- **Squamous cells:** Thin, flat cells that form the top layer of the epidermis.

- **Basal cells:** Round cells under the squamous cells.

- **Melanocytes:** Cells that make melanin and are found in the lower part of the epidermis. Melanin is the pigment that gives skin its natural color. When skin is exposed to the sun or artificial light, melanocytes make more pigment and cause the skin to darken.

The number of new cases of melanoma has been increasing over the last 40 years. Melanoma is most common in adults, but it is sometimes found in children and adolescents.

Types Of Skin Cancer

There are two forms of skin cancer: Melanoma and Nonmelanoma.

Melanoma is a rare form of skin cancer. It is more likely to invade nearby tissues and spread to other parts of the body than other types of skin cancer. When melanoma starts in the skin, it is called cutaneous melanoma. Melanoma may also occur in mucous membranes (thin, moist layers of tissue that cover surfaces such as the lips).

The most common types of skin cancer are basal cell carcinoma and squamous cell carcinoma. They are nonmelanoma skin cancers. Nonmelanoma skin cancers rarely spread to other parts of the body.

Melanoma Can Occur Anywhere On The Skin

In men, melanoma is often found on the trunk (the area from the shoulders to the hips) or the head and neck. In women, melanoma forms most often on the arms and legs.

When melanoma occurs in the eye, it is called intraocular or ocular melanoma.

The Risk Of Melanoma

Unusual Moles, exposure to sunlight, and health history can affect the risk of melanoma.

Anything that increases your risk of getting a disease is called a risk factor. Having a risk factor does not mean that you will get cancer; not having risk factors doesn't **mean that you will not get cancer. Talk with your doctor if you think you may be at risk.**

Risk factors for melanoma include the following:

- Having a fair complexion, which includes the following:
  - Fair skin that freckles and burns easily, does not tan, or tans poorly.
  - Blue or green or other light-colored eyes.
  - Red or blond hair.
- Being exposed to natural sunlight or artificial sunlight (such as from tanning beds) over long periods of time.
- Being exposed to certain factors in the environment (in the air, your home or workplace, and your food and water). Some of the environmental risk factors for melanoma are radiation, solvents, vinyl chloride, and PCBs.
- Having a history of many blistering sunburns, especially as a child or teenager.
- Having several large or many small moles.
- Having a family history of unusual moles (atypical nevus syndrome).
- Having a family or personal history of melanoma.
- Being white.
- Having a weakened immune system.
- Having certain changes in the genes that are linked to melanoma.

Being white or having a fair complexion increases the risk of melanoma, but anyone can have melanoma, including people with dark skin.

Signs Of Melanoma

Signs of melanoma include a change in the way a mole or pigmented area looks.

These and other signs and symptoms may be caused by melanoma or by other conditions.

Check with your doctor if you have any of the following:

- A mole that:

  - changes in size, shape, or color.

  - has irregular edges or borders.

  - is more than one color.

  - is asymmetrical (if the mole is divided in half, the 2 halves are different in size or shape).

  - itches.

  - oozes, bleeds, or is ulcerated (a hole forms in the skin when the top layer of cells breaks down and the tissue below shows through).

  - A change in pigmented (colored) skin.

  - Satellite moles (new moles that grow near an existing mole).

Tests That Examine The Skin Are Used To Detect (Find) And Diagnose Melanoma

If a mole or pigmented area of the skin changes or looks abnormal, the following tests and procedures can help find and diagnose melanoma:

- **Skin exam:** A doctor or nurse checks the skin for moles, birthmarks, or other pigmented areas that look abnormal in color, size, shape, or texture.

- **Biopsy:** A procedure to remove the abnormal tissue and a small amount of normal tissue around it. A pathologist looks at the tissue under a microscope to check for cancer cells. It can be hard to tell the difference between a colored mole and an early melanoma lesion. Patients may want to have the sample of tissue checked by a second pathologist. If the abnormal mole or lesion is cancer, the sample of tissue may also be tested for certain gene changes.

It is important that abnormal areas of the skin not be shaved off or cauterized (destroyed with a hot instrument, an electric current, or a caustic substance) because cancer cells that remain may grow and spread.

Certain Factors Affect Prognosis (Chance Of Recovery) And Treatment Options

The prognosis (chance of recovery) and treatment options depend on the following:

- The thickness of the tumor and where it is in the body.

- How quickly the cancer cells are dividing.

- Whether there was bleeding or ulceration of the tumor.

- How much cancer is in the lymph nodes.

- The number of places cancer has spread to in the body.

- The level of lactate dehydrogenase (LDH) in the blood.

- Whether the cancer has certain mutations (changes) in a gene called BRAF.

- The patient's age and general health.

Treatment Options For Actinic Keratosis[1]

Actinic keratosis is not cancer but is treated because it may develop into cancer. Treatment of actinic keratosis may include the following:

- Topical chemotherapy

- Topical biologic therapy with imiquimod

- Cryosurgery

- Electrodesiccation and curettage

- Dermabrasion

- Shave excision

- Photodynamic therapy

- Laser surgery

Chapter 32

Common Moles And Dysplastic Nevi

What Is A Common Mole?

A common mole is a growth on the skin that develops when pigment cells (melanocytes) grow in clusters. These growths are usually found above the waist on areas exposed to the sun. They are seldom found on the scalp, breast, or buttocks.

Although common moles may be present at birth, they usually appear later in childhood. Most people continue to develop new moles until about age 40. In older people, common moles tend to fade away.

Another name for a mole is a nevus. The plural is nevi.

What Does A Common Mole Look Like?

A common mole is usually smaller than about 5 millimeters wide (about 1/4 inch, the width of a pencil eraser). It is round or oval, has a smooth surface with a distinct edge, and is often dome-shaped. A common mole usually has an even color of pink, tan, or brown. People who have dark skin or hair tend to have darker moles than people with fair skin or blonde hair.

What Is A Dysplastic Nevus?

A dysplastic nevus is a type of mole that looks different from a common mole. (Some doctors use the term "atypical mole" to refer to a dysplastic nevus.) A dysplastic nevus may be

About This Chapter: This chapter includes text excerpted from "Common Moles, Dysplastic Nevi, And Risk Of Melanoma," National Cancer Institute (NCI),May 3, 2017.

bigger than a common mole, and its color, surface, and border may be different. It is usually more than 5 millimeters wide. A dysplastic nevus can have a mixture of several colors, from pink to dark brown. Usually, it is flat with a smooth, slightly scaly, or pebbly surface, and it has an irregular edge that may fade into the surrounding skin.

A dysplastic nevus may occur anywhere on the body, but it is usually seen in areas exposed to the sun, such as on the back. A dysplastic nevus may also appear in areas not exposed to the sun, such as the scalp, breasts, and areas below the waist. Some people have only a couple of dysplastic nevi, but other people have more than 10. People who have dysplastic nevi usually also have an increased number of common moles.

What Should People Do If They Have A Dysplastic Nevus?

Everyone should protect their skin from the sun and stay away from sunlamps and tanning booths, but for people who have dysplastic nevi, it is even more important to protect the skin and avoid getting a suntan or sunburn.

In addition, many doctors recommend that people with dysplastic nevi check their skin once a month. People should tell their doctor if they see any of the following changes in a dysplastic nevus:

- The color changes

- It gets smaller or bigger

- It changes in shape, texture, or height

- The skin on the surface becomes dry or scaly

- It becomes hard or feels lumpy

- It starts to itch

- It bleeds or oozes

Another thing that people with dysplastic nevi should do is get their skin examined by a doctor. Sometimes people or their doctors take photographs of dysplastic nevi so changes over time are easier to see. For people with many (more than five) dysplastic nevi, doctors may conduct a skin exam once or twice a year because of the moderately increased chance of melanoma. For people who also have a family history of melanoma, doctors may suggest a more frequent skin exam, such as every 3 to 6 months.

Should People Have A Doctor Remove A Dysplastic Nevus Or A Common Mole?

No. Normally, people do not need to have a dysplastic nevus or common mole removed. One reason is that very few dysplastic nevi or common moles turn into melanoma. Another reason is that even removing all of the moles on the skin would not prevent the development of melanoma because melanoma can develop as a new colored area on the skin. That is why doctors usually remove only a mole that changes or a new colored area on the skin.

What Are The Differences Between A Common Mole And A Dysplastic Nevus?

Common moles and dysplastic nevi vary by size, color, shape, and surface texture. The list below summarizes some differences between them.

Common Mole (Nevus)

- **Is it cancer?** No. Common moles rarely become cancer.

- **How big are they?** Usually less than 5 millimeters wide, or about 1/4 inch (not as wide as a new pencil eraser).

- **What color are they?** May be pink, tan, brown, black (in people with dark skin), or a color that is very close to a person's normal skin tone. The color is usually even throughout.

- **What shape are they?** Usually round or oval. A common mole has a distinct edge that separates it from the rest of the skin.

- **What is the surface texture?** Begins as a flat, smooth spot on the skin. May become raised and form a smooth bump.

Dysplastic Nevus

- **Is it cancer?** No. A dysplastic nevus is more likely than a common mole to become cancer, but most do not become cancer.

- **How big are they?** Often wider than 5 millimeters (wider than a new pencil eraser).

- **What color are they?** May be a mixture of tan, brown, and red or pink shades.

- **What shape are they?** Have irregular or notched edges. May fade into the rest of the skin.

- **What is the surface texture?** May have a smooth, slightly scaly, or rough, irregular, and pebbly appearance.

What Should People Do If A Mole Changes, Or They Find A New Mole Or Some Other Change On Their Skin?

People should tell their doctor if they find a new mole or a change in an existing mole. A family doctor may refer people with an unusual mole or other concerns about their skin to a dermatologist. A dermatologist is a doctor who specializes in diseases of the skin. Also, some plastic surgeons, general surgeons, internists, cancer specialists, and family doctors have special training in moles.

Chapter 33

Pruritus (Itching)

Pruritus is an itchy feeling that makes you want to scratch your skin. It may occur without a rash or skin lesions. Pruritus sometimes feels like pain because the signals for itching and pain travel along the same nerve pathways. Scratching may cause breaks in the skin, bleeding, and infection. If your skin feels itchy, let your doctor know so it can be treated and relieved.

The way pruritus feels and how long it lasts is not the same in everyone.

The skin is the largest organ of the body. The most important job of skin is to protect against heat, sunlight, injury, and infection. The skin is also important to self-image and your ability to touch and be touched.

Certain conditions, cancers, and blood disorders may cause pruritus.

Pruritus is a symptom of a certain condition, blood disorder, or a disease. These include:

- Cancer and conditions related to cancer.

- Liver, kidney, or thyroid disorders.

- Diabetes mellitus.

- Human immunodeficiency virus (HIV) or parasite infection.

- Dry skin.

- Drug reactions.

- Conditions related to stress, anxiety, or depression.

The cause of pruritus is not always known.

About This Chapter: This chapter includes text excerpted from "Pruritus (PDQ®)—Patient Version," National Cancer Institute (NCI), June 15, 2016.

Causes Of Pruritus

Certain Cancer Treatments May Cause Pruritus

Cancer treatments that may cause pruritus include chemotherapy, radiation therapy, and immunotherapy (biologic therapy).

- When chemotherapy causes pruritus, it may be a sign that you are sensitive to the drugs being used.

- Radiation therapy can kill skin cells and cause dryness, burning, and itching as the skin peels off.

- Drugs used in immunotherapy may also cause dryness and itching.

Skin can become thin and dry because many of these therapies make your skin less able to make new cells and heal. Long-term dry skin may occur when hair and sweat gland function does not return to normal right after cancer treatment.

Drugs May Be Used For Supportive Care

Some of the drugs used to prevent or treat cancer symptoms may cause pruritus, including the following:

- Pain medicine such as opioids

- Drugs for nausea and vomiting

- Hormones such as estrogens, testosterone, or progestins

Assessment Of Pruritus

Finding the cause of the itching is the first step in relieving pruritus.

Since pruritus is a symptom of a disease or condition, finding and treating the cause is the first step in bringing you relief.

A physical exam, blood tests, and a chest X-ray are done to assess pruritus.

The following tests and procedures may be done to find the problem that is causing the itching:

- Physical exam and history

- Blood chemistry studies

- Complete blood count (CBC) with differential

- Sedimentation rate

- Chest X-ray

Depending on the results, further tests, such as a skin biopsy, may be done to diagnose the problem and decide on treatment.

Treatment Of Pruritus

Treatment of pruritus in cancer patients involves learning what the triggers are and taking steps to avoid them.

It is important for you and for caregivers to know what triggers itching, such as dry skin or hot baths, so you can take steps to prevent it. You may need more than one type of treatment to relieve or prevent pruritus, protect your skin, and keep you comfortable.

Good nutrition is very important for healthy skin. A good diet includes a balance of proteins, carbohydrates, fats, vitamins, minerals, and fluids. Eating a balanced diet and drinking plenty of fluids helps your skin stay healthy. It is best to drink at least 3 liters (about 100 ounces) of fluid each day, but this may not be possible for everyone.

Washing the skin every day or every two days is important to help remove dirt and keep the skin healthy.

Different Types Of Treatment Are Used To Help Treat Pruritus

Self-Care

Self-care includes avoiding pruritus triggers and taking good care of your skin.

Pruritus triggers include:

- Dehydration caused by fever, diarrhea, nausea and vomiting, or low fluid intake.

- Hot baths or bathing more than once a day, or for longer than 30 minutes.

- Bubble baths or soaps with detergents.

- Reusable scrubbing sponges for the face or loofahs for the body.

- Scents, fragrances, and perfumes.

- Adding oil at the beginning of the bath.

- Dry indoor air.

- Laundry detergent with scents, dyes, or preservatives.

- Fabric softener sheets.

- Tight clothes or clothes made of wool, synthetics, or other harsh/scratchy fabric.

- Underarm deodorants or antiperspirants.

- Skin care or cosmetics with scents, dyes, or preservatives.

- Emotional stress.

Ways to help lessen itching include:

- Using unscented, soothing creams or ointments.

- Bathing in slightly warm water no more than 30 minutes daily or every other day.

- Using mild skin cleansers (nonsoap) or soaps made for sensitive skin (such as Cetaphil cleanser, Dove for Sensitive Skin, Oilatum, Basis).

- Adding oil and soap at the end of a bath or adding a colloidal oatmeal treatment early to the bath.

- Using soap only for dirty areas; otherwise water is good enough.

- Gently washing, if needed, with a clean, fresh, soft cotton washcloth.

- Rinsing all soap or other residue from bathing with fresh, slightly warm water.

- Drying off by patting skin instead of rubbing.

- Keeping home air cool and humid (including use of a humidifier).

- Washing sheets, clothes, and underwear in mild soap or baby soap that contains no scents, dyes, or preservatives (such as Dreft, All Free Clear, Tide Free and Gentle). Adding vinegar (one teaspoon per quart of water) to rinse water removes traces of detergent.

- Using liquid fabric softener that gets rinsed out in the wash (such as All Free Clear Fabric Softener) or avoiding fabric softener altogether.

- Using blankets that are soft, such as cotton flannel.

- Wearing loose-fitting clothes and clothes made of cotton or other soft fabrics.

- Using distraction, music therapy, relaxation, or positive imagery.

Over-The-Counter Treatments

Some over-the-counter treatments (medicines that can be bought without a prescription) help prevent or relieve pruritus. However, you should read labels carefully to look for ingredients that may trigger skin reactions, including alcohol, topical antibiotics, and topical anesthetics.

Cornstarch And Talc

Cornstarch can help prevent itching of dry skin caused by radiation therapy but should not be used where skin is moist. When cornstarch becomes moist, fungus may grow. Avoid using it on areas close to mucous membranes, such as the vagina or rectum, in skin folds, and on areas that have hair or sweat glands.

Some powders and antiperspirants, such as those that contain talc and aluminum, cause skin irritation during radiation therapy and should be avoided when you're receiving radiation treatment.

For itching not related to radiation therapy, talc-based treatments may be better than cornstarch-based treatments, especially where two skin surfaces touch or rub together (such as the underarm or between fingers or toes).

Creams And Lotions

If pruritus is related to dry skin, emollient creams or lotions may be used. Emollients help soothe and soften the skin and increase moisture levels in the skin. It is important to know the ingredients in these creams and lotions because some may cause skin reactions. Such ingredients include:

- Petrolatum, which is not well absorbed in skin treated with radiation therapy and may buildup too much or be hard to remove.

- Lanolin, which may cause allergic reactions in some people.

- Mineral oil, which may be combined with petrolatum and lanolin in creams and lotions and may be an ingredient in bath oils.

Other ingredients added to emollients, such as thickeners, preservatives, fragrances, and colorings, may also cause allergic skin reactions.

Emollient creams or lotions are applied at least two or three times a day and after bathing. Gels with a local anesthetic (0.5%–5% lidocaine) can be used on some small areas as often as every 2 hours if you aren't sensitive to alcohol ingredients.

To soothe or cool areas of severe pruritus, over-the-counter products containing menthol, camphor, pramoxine, or capsaicin can be used. These products soothe, cool, and decrease the urge to scratch. Capsaicin-based therapies may work best in pruritus related to nerve signals.

Prescription Drugs Applied To The Skin

Your doctor may prescribe topical steroids (steroids applied to the skin) to reduce itching, but they cause thinning of the skin and make it more sensitive. They should be used only for pruritus related to inflammation. Topical steroids should not be used on skin being treated with radiation therapy, but may be used to relieve inflamed skin after radiation treatment ends.

For xerosis (abnormally dry skin) or keratoderma (a horn-like skin condition), moisturizer creams may be used to seal in moisture and peel off scaly layers of skin. Humectants with ingredients like salicylic acid, ammonium lactate, or urea may improve skin smoothness but can cause stinging if applied to broken skin.

Systemic Therapies

Systemic therapies travel through the bloodstream and reach and affect cells all over the body. They may help treat the condition causing your pruritus or help control your symptoms.

Your doctor may prescribe an antibiotic if your pruritus is caused by an infection. You may also be given an oral antihistamine to relieve itching. A larger dose may sometimes be used at bedtime to help you sleep.

Other Drug Therapies

If other drug treatments do not work to control pruritus, sedatives and antidepressants are sometimes used.

Aspirin may relieve pruritus in some patients with polycythemia vera but may increase pruritus in others. Cimetidine alone or combined with aspirin may help control pruritus in patients with Hodgkin lymphoma and polycythemia vera.

Comfort Measures

Other steps may be taken to help you keep from scratching and stop the itch-scratch-itch cycle. These may include:

- Applying emollients to help prevent skin breakdown.
- A cool washcloth or ice held over the itchy area.
- Firm pressure on the itchy area, on the same area on the opposite side of the body, and at acupressure points.
- Rubbing or vibration on the itchy area.
- Transcutaneous electrical nerve stimulation (TENS) or acupuncture.

Chapter 34

Psoriasis

What Is Psoriasis?

Psoriasis is a chronic (long-lasting) skin disease of scaling and inflammation that affects greater than 3.1 percent of the U.S. population, or more than 6.7 million adults. Although the disease occurs in all age groups, it primarily affects adults. It appears about equally in males and females.

Psoriasis occurs when skin cells quickly rise from their origin below the surface of the skin and pile up on the surface before they have a chance to mature. Usually this movement (also called turnover) takes about a month, but in psoriasis it may occur in only a few days.

In its typical form, psoriasis results in patches of thick, red (inflamed) skin covered with silvery scales. These patches, which are sometimes referred to as plaques, usually itch or feel sore. They most often occur on the elbows, knees, other parts of the legs, scalp, lower back, face, palms, and soles of the feet, but they can occur on skin anywhere on the body. The disease may also affect the fingernails, the toenails, and the soft tissues of the genitals, and inside the mouth.

How Does Psoriasis Affect Quality Of Life?

Individuals with psoriasis may experience significant physical discomfort and some disability. Itching and pain can interfere with basic functions, such as self-care, walking, and sleep. Plaques on hands and feet can prevent individuals from working at certain occupations,

About This Chapter: This chapter includes text excerpted from "Psoriasis—Questions And Answers About Psoriasis," National Institute of Arthritis and Musculoskeletal and Skin Diseases (NIAMS), March 2017.

playing some sports, and caring for family members or a home. The frequency of medical care is costly and can interfere with an employment or school schedule. People with moderate to severe psoriasis may feel self-conscious about their appearance. Psychological distress can lead to depression and social isolation.

What Causes Psoriasis?

Psoriasis is a skin disorder driven by the immune system, especially involving a type of white blood cell called a T cell. Normally, T cells help protect the body against infection and disease. In the case of psoriasis, T cells are put into action by mistake and become so active that they trigger other immune responses, which lead to inflammation and to rapid turnover of skin cells.

In many cases, there is a family history of psoriasis. Researchers have studied a large number of families affected by psoriasis and identified genes linked to the disease.

People with psoriasis may notice that there are times when their skin worsens, called flares, then improves. Conditions that may cause flares include infections, stress, and changes in climate that dry the skin. Also, certain medicines may trigger an outbreak or worsen the disease. Sometimes people who have psoriasis notice that lesions will appear where the skin has experienced trauma. The trauma could be from a cut, scratch, sunburn, or infection.

Avoid Psoriasis Triggers

Factors that may trigger psoriasis or make it worse include:

- physical and emotional stress
- injury to the skin such as cuts or burns
- infections, especially strep throat
- cold weather
- smoking or heavy alcohol use

(Source: "Spotlight On Psoriasis," NIH News in Health, National Institutes of Health (NIH).)

How Is Psoriasis Diagnosed?

Occasionally, doctors may find it difficult to diagnose psoriasis, because it often looks like other skin diseases. It may be necessary to confirm a diagnosis by examining a small skin sample under a microscope.

There are several forms of psoriasis. Some of these include:

- **Plaque psoriasis.** Skin lesions are red at the base and covered by silvery scales.

- **Guttate psoriasis.** Small, drop-shaped lesions appear on the trunk, limbs, and scalp. Guttate psoriasis is most often triggered by upper respiratory infections (for example, a sore throat caused by streptococcal bacteria).

- **Pustular psoriasis.** Blisters of noninfectious pus appear on the skin. Attacks of pustular psoriasis may be triggered by medications, infections, stress, or exposure to certain chemicals.

- **Inverse psoriasis.** Smooth, red patches occur in the folds of the skin near the genitals, under the breasts, or in the armpits. The symptoms may be worsened by friction and sweating.

- **Erythrodermic psoriasis.** Widespread reddening and scaling of the skin may be a reaction to severe sunburn or to taking corticosteroids (cortisone) or other medications. It can also be caused by a prolonged period of increased activity of psoriasis that is poorly controlled. Erythrodermic psoriasis can be very serious and requires immediate medical attention.

Another condition in which people may experience psoriasis is **psoriatic arthritis.** This is a form of arthritis that produces the joint inflammation common in arthritis and the lesions common in psoriasis. The joint inflammation and the skin lesions don't necessarily have to occur at the same time.

How Is Psoriasis Treated?

Doctors generally treat psoriasis in steps based on the severity of the disease, size of the areas involved, type of psoriasis, where the psoriasis is located, and the patient's response to initial treatments. Treatment can include:

- medicines applied to the skin (topical treatment)

- light treatment (phototherapy)

- medicines by mouth or injection (systemic therapy).

Over time, affected skin can become resistant to treatment, especially when topical corticosteroids are used. Also, a treatment that works very well in one person may have little effect in another. Thus, doctors often use a trial-and-error approach to find a treatment that works, and they may switch treatments periodically if a treatment does not work or if adverse reactions occur.

Topical Treatment

Treatments applied directly to the skin may improve its condition. Doctors find that some patients respond well to ointment or cream forms of corticosteroids, vitamin D3, retinoids, coal tar, or anthralin. Bath solutions and lubricants may be soothing, but they are seldom strong enough to improve the condition of the skin. Therefore, they usually are combined with stronger remedies.

Light Therapy

Natural ultraviolet (UV) light from the sun and controlled delivery of artificial UV light are used in treating psoriasis. It is important that light therapy be administered by a doctor. Spending time in the sun or a tanning bed can cause skin damage, increase the risk of skin cancer, and worsen symptoms.

Systemic Treatment

For more severe forms of psoriasis, doctors sometimes prescribe medicines that are taken internally by pill or injection. This is called systemic treatment.

- **Retinoids.** Oral retinoids are compounds with vitamin A-like properties that may be prescribed for severe cases of psoriasis that do not respond to other therapies. Because these medications also may cause birth defects, women must protect themselves from pregnancy.

- **Cyclosporine.** Taken orally, cyclosporine acts by suppressing the immune system to slow the rapid turnover of skin cells. It may provide quick relief of symptoms, but the improvement stops when treatment is discontinued. Cyclosporine may impair kidney function or cause high blood pressure (hypertension). Therefore, patients must be carefully monitored by a doctor.

- **Methotrexate.** Like cyclosporine, methotrexate slows cell turnover by suppressing the immune system. It can be taken by pill or injection. Patients taking methotrexate must be closely monitored because it can cause liver damage and/or decrease the production of oxygen-carrying red blood cells, infection-fighting white blood cells, and clot-enhancing platelets.

- **PDE4 inhibitors**. Taken orally, phosphodiesterase 4 (PDE4) inhibitors target molecules inside immune cells to suppress the rapid turnover of skin cells and inflammation.

- **Biologic response modifiers.** Biologics are made from proteins produced by living cells instead of chemicals. They interfere with specific immune system processes which cause the overproduction of skin cells and inflammation. These drugs are injected (sometimes by the patient). Patients taking these treatments need to be monitored carefully by a doctor. Because these drugs suppress the immune system response, patients taking these drugs have an increased risk of infection, and the drugs may also interfere with patients taking vaccines. Also, some of these drugs have been associated with other diseases (like central nervous system disorders, blood diseases, cancer, and lymphoma) although their role in the development of or contribution to these diseases is not yet understood.

Combination Therapy

Combining various topical, light, and systemic treatments often permits lower doses of each and can result in increased effectiveness. There are many approaches for treating psoriasis. Ask the doctor about the best options for you. Find out:

- How long the treatment may last.

- How long it will take to see results.

- What the possible side effects are.

- What to do if the side effects are severe.

Chapter 35

Pyogenic Granuloma And Pityriasis Rosea

Pyogenic Granuloma

Pyogenic granuloma, also called lobular capillary hemangioma, is a benign (noncancerous) skin growth that looks like a small, raised, red bump. These growths usually appear on the face, neck, hands, upper trunk, and feet. They also contain numerous blood vessels so will tend to bleed easily. While most commonly found in children and teens, pyogenic granuloma can occur at any age. The condition is also common in pregnant women, but the growths generally appear in the mouth.

Causes

The actual cause for pyogenic granuloma is unknown. However, pyogenic granuloma generally occurs after a minor injury and can grow rapidly within a few weeks to over half an inch.

Treatment

A healthcare provider would first diagnose the condition based on a physical examination. A skin biopsy may also be necessary in rare cases to rule out the possibility of cancer. Smaller pyogenic granuloma can disappear without treatment. However larger bumps need to be treated. The most common procedure is to scrape the growth off the skin using an instrument called a curette, then lightly cauterize (sear) the wound to prevent bleeding and further growth. Doctors may also freeze and remove the growth, use laser surgery, or apply certain chemicals, such as silver nitrate, phenol, or podophyllin. Cure rates are higher when the bump is completely removed and closed with stitches. However, the growth may recur if it is not completely removed. Pregnant women may find pyogenic granuloma disappear without treatment after their pregnancy.

Pityriasis Rosea

Pityriasis rosea is a common skin disease characterized by a reddish, scaly rash that lasts for several weeks or months. A large patch called "mother patch" or "herald patch" appears first and remains for about 2 weeks. This is followed by smaller patches called "daughter patches" appearing on the chest, abdomen, arms, and legs that remain active for 6–8 weeks. Pityriasis rosea mostly affects people between the ages of 10 and 35, but can occur at any age. The condition requires no treatment and is not contagious.

Causes

The exact cause of pityriasis rosea is unknown. It is not an allergic reaction nor is it caused by a fungus or bacteria. However, some researchers believe that it may be caused by certain type of herpes virus.

Symptoms

A large patch that is pink in color, oval or round in shape, and 2 cm to 10 cm in size appears first and remains on the skin for two weeks. You may also feel tired and achy (as if you are catching a cold) just before this first patch appears.

Following the appearance of the first patch, a number of small salmon-colored patches appear commonly on the chest, arms, legs, and abdomen. They might also appear on the neck, face, and elsewhere on the skin. When many patches appear, they may form a pattern like the shape of a Christmas tree.

The patches may make the skin itch. The itch can become intense when the skin is warm, such as when a person takes a hot shower or exercises.

Diagnosis

The healthcare provider would be able to diagnose pityriasis rosea by physical examination. When only the herald patch is present, doctors may mistake the condition for eczema or ringworm. To rule out other possible conditions that appear similar, other tests may be done, including:

- A potassium hydroxide (KOH) test to ensure the rash is not of fungal origin.

- A biopsy to rule out any possibility of cancer.

- A syphilis test if the patient is sexually active.

Treatment

There is no specific treatment recommended for pityriasis rosea and it usually goes away on its own. However, your healthcare provider will likely focus any treatment on relieving the itching associated with the rash. Treatment may include:

- Anti-inflammatories (Corticosteroids)

- Antihistamines such as chlorpheniramine maleate (Chlor-Trimeton)

- Diphenhydramine (Benadryl). This is not recommended for children unless prescribed by a healthcare provider

Those suffering from pityraisis rosea can also minimize any discomfort by taking the following steps:

- Dress coolly and avoid getting overheated

- Avoid hot showers and baths. Use only lukewarm water.

- Take an oatmeal bath.

- Use only mild soaps, such as cetaphil or dove.

- Use an over-the-counter 1percent hydrocortisone cream as directed.

References

1. "Pyogenic Granuloma," National Institutes of Health (NIH), July 5, 2017.

2. "Pyogenic Granuloma," American Osteopathic College of Dermatology (AOCD), n.d.

3. Eleni, Yiasemides. "Pyogenic Granuloma," The Australasian College of Dermatologists, n.d.

4. "Pityriasis Rosea," American Osteopathic College of Dermatology (AOCD), n.d.

5. "Pityriasis Rosea—Topic Overview," Web MD, n.d.

6. "Pityriasis Rosea," American Academy of Dermatology (AAD), n.d.

7. "Diseases And Conditions—Pityriasis Rosea," Mayo Clinic, n.d.

Chapter 36

Rosacea

What Is Rosacea?

Rosacea is a chronic (long-term) disease that affects the skin and sometimes the eyes. The disorder is characterized by redness, pimples, and, in advanced stages, thickened skin. Rosacea usually affects the face. Skin on other parts of the upper body is only rarely involved.

Who Gets Rosacea?

Rosacea most often affects middle-age and older adults. It is more common in women (particularly during menopause) than men. Although rosacea can develop in people of any skin color, it tends to occur most frequently and is most apparent in people with fair skin.

What Are The Symptoms Of Rosacea?

There are several symptoms and conditions associated with rosacea. These include frequent flushing, vascular rosacea, inflammatory rosacea, and several other conditions involving the skin, eyes, and nose.

Frequent flushing of the center of the face, which may include the forehead, nose, cheeks, and chin, occurs in the earliest stage of rosacea. The flushing often is accompanied by a burning sensation, particularly when creams or cosmetics are applied to the face. Sometimes the face is swollen slightly.

About This Chapter: This chapter includes text excerpted from "Rosacea—Questions And Answers About Rosacea," National Institute of Arthritis and Musculoskeletal and Skin Diseases (NIAMS), April 2016.

A condition called vascular rosacea causes persistent flushing and redness. Blood vessels under the skin of the face may dilate (enlarge), showing through the skin as small red lines. This is called telangiectasia. The affected skin may be swollen slightly and feel warm.

A condition called inflammatory rosacea causes persistent redness and papules (pink bumps) and pustules (bumps containing pus) on the skin. Eye inflammation and sensitivity as well as telangiectasia also may occur.

In the most advanced stage of rosacea, the skin becomes a deep shade of red and inflammation of the eye is more apparent. Numerous telangiectases are often present, and nodules in the skin may become painful. A condition called rhinophyma also may develop in some men; it is rare in women. Rhinophyma is characterized by an enlarged, bulbous, and red nose resulting from enlargement of the sebaceous (oil-producing) glands beneath the surface of the skin on the nose. People who have rosacea also may develop a thickening of the skin on the forehead, chin, cheeks, or other areas.

In addition to skin problems, many people who have rosacea have eye problems caused by the condition. Typical symptoms include redness, dryness, itching, burning, tearing, and the sensation of having sand in the eye. The eyelids may become inflamed and swollen. Some people say their eyes are sensitive to light and their vision is blurred or otherwise impaired.

What Causes Rosacea?

Doctors do not know the exact cause of rosacea but believe that some people may inherit a tendency to develop the disorder. People who blush frequently may be more likely to develop rosacea. Some researchers believe that rosacea is a disorder where blood vessels dilate too easily, resulting in flushing and redness.

Factors that cause rosacea to flare up in one person may have no effect on another person. Although the following factors have not been well-researched, some people claim that one or more of them have aggravated their rosacea: heat (including hot baths), strenuous exercise, sunlight, wind, very cold temperatures, hot or spicy foods and drinks, alcohol consumption, menopause, emotional stress, long-term use of topical steroids on the face, and bacteria.

How Is Rosacea Treated?

Although there is no cure for rosacea, it can be treated and controlled. A dermatologist (a medical doctor who specializes in diseases of the skin) usually treats rosacea. The goals of treatment are to control the condition and improve the appearance of the patient's skin. It may take several weeks or months of treatment before a person notices an improvement of the skin.

Treatments for rosacea include medicines that are applied directly to the affected skin. Some doctors will prescribe a topical antibiotic, which is applied directly to the affected skin. For people with more severe cases, doctors may prescribe an oral (taken by mouth) antibiotic.

Patients can play an important role in managing rosacea. You can take several steps to keep rosacea under control:

- Keep a written record of when flares occur. This may provide clues about what is irritating the skin.

- Use sunscreen. Most people should use a sunscreen every day that protects against ultraviolet A (UVA) and ultraviolet B (UVB) rays and has a sun-protection factor (SPF) of 15 or higher, but sunscreen is particularly important for people whose skin is irritated by exposure to the sun.

- Use a mild lubricant if you find it is helpful, but avoid applying any irritating products to the face. Some people find that a green-tinted makeup effectively conceals skin redness.

Doctors usually treat the eye problems of rosacea with prescription eye medicine. People who develop infections of the eyelids must practice frequent eyelid hygiene. The doctor may recommend scrubbing the eyelids gently with diluted baby shampoo or an over-the-counter eyelid cleaner and applying warm (but not hot) compresses several times a day. Electrosurgery, dermabrasion, and laser surgery may be used if red lines caused by dilated blood vessels appear in the skin or if skin thickening develops.

Ask the doctor about how to manage rosacea and what treatment options are best for you. A combination of treatments may work best. Find out:

- How long the treatment may last.

- How long it will take to see results.

- What the possible side effects are.

- What you should do if the side effects are severe.

Chapter 37

Scleroderma

What Is Scleroderma?

Derived from the Greek words "*sklerosis*," meaning hardness, and "derma," meaning skin, scleroderma literally means "hard skin." Although it is often referred to as if it were a single disease, scleroderma is really a symptom of a group of diseases that involve the abnormal growth of connective tissue, which supports the skin and internal organs. In some forms of scleroderma, hard, tight skin is the extent of this abnormal process. In other forms, however, the problem goes much deeper, affecting blood vessels and internal organs, such as the heart, lungs, and kidneys.

Scleroderma is called both a rheumatic disease and a connective tissue disease. The term rheumatic disease refers to a group of conditions characterized by inflammation or pain in the muscles, joints, or fibrous tissue. A connective tissue disease is one that affects tissues such as skin, tendons, and cartilage.

Scleroderma is also believed to be an autoimmune disease. In autoimmune diseases, the body's immune system turns against and damages its own tissues.

What Are The Different Types Of Scleroderma?

The group of diseases we call scleroderma falls into two main classes: localized scleroderma and systemic sclerosis. (Localized diseases affect only certain parts of the body; systemic diseases can affect the whole body.) Both groups include subgroups. Although there are different ways these groups and subgroups may be broken down or referred to (and your doctor may use different terms from what you see here), the following is a common way of classifying these diseases:

About This Chapter: This chapter includes text excerpted from "Scleroderma—Handout On Health: Scleroderma," National Institute of Arthritis and Musculoskeletal and Skin Diseases (NIAMS), August 2016.

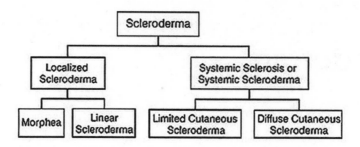

Figure 37.1. Types Of Scleroderma

Localized Scleroderma

Localized types of scleroderma are those limited to the skin and related tissues and, in some cases, the muscle below. Internal organs are not affected by localized scleroderma, and localized scleroderma can never progress to the systemic form of the disease. Often, localized conditions improve or go away on their own over time, but the skin changes and damage that occur when the disease is active can be permanent. For some people, localized scleroderma is serious and disabling.

There are two generally recognized types of localized scleroderma:

Morphea: Morphea refers to local patches of scleroderma. The first signs of the disease are reddish patches of skin that thicken into firm, oval-shaped areas. Patches appear most often on the chest, stomach, and back. Sometimes they appear on the face, arms, and legs.

Morphea can be either localized or generalized. *Localized morphea* limits itself to one or several patches, ranging in size from a half-inch to 12 inches in diameter. Some people have both morphea and linear scleroderma. The disease is referred to as *generalized morphea* when the skin patches become very hard and dark and spread over larger areas of the body. Regardless of the type, morphea generally fades out in 3 to 5 years; however, people are often left with darkened skin patches and, in rare cases, muscle weakness.

Linear scleroderma: As suggested by its name, the disease is characterized by a single line or band of thickened or abnormally colored skin. Usually, the line runs down an arm or leg, but in some people it runs down the forehead.

Systemic Scleroderma (Also Known As Systemic Sclerosis)

This is the term for the form of the disease that not only includes the skin, but also involves the tissues beneath, the blood vessels, and the major organs. Systemic sclerosis is typically broken down into *limited cutaneous scleroderma* and *diffuse cutaneous scleroderma*.

Limited cutaneous scleroderma: Limited cutaneous scleroderma typically comes on gradually and affects the skin only in certain areas: the fingers, hands, face, lower arms, and legs. People with limited disease often have all or some of the symptoms that some doctors call CREST, which stands for the following:

- **Calcinosis:** The formation of calcium deposits in the connective tissues, which can be detected by X-ray.

- **Raynaud phenomenon:** A condition in which the small blood vessels of the hands or feet contract in response to cold or anxiety.

- **Esophageal dysfunction:** Impaired function of the esophagus (the tube connecting the throat and the stomach) that occurs when smooth muscles in the esophagus lose normal movement.

- **Sclerodactyly:** Thick and tight skin on the fingers, resulting from deposits of excess collagen within skin layers.

- **Telangiectasia:** A condition caused by the swelling of tiny blood vessels, in which small red spots appear on the hands and face.

Diffuse cutaneous scleroderma: This condition typically comes on suddenly. Skin thickening begins in the hands and spreads quickly and over much of the body, affecting the hands, face, upper arms, upper legs, chest, and stomach in a symmetrical fashion (for example, if one arm or one side of the trunk is affected, the other is also affected). Some people may have more area of their skin affected than others. Internally, this condition can damage key organs such as the intestines, lungs, heart, and kidneys.

People with diffuse scleroderma face the most serious long-term outlook if they develop severe kidney, lung, digestive, or heart problems. Fortunately, less than one-third of patients with diffuse disease develop these severe problems. Early diagnosis and continual and careful monitoring are important.

What Causes Scleroderma?

Although scientists don't know exactly what causes scleroderma, they are certain that people cannot catch it from or transmit it to others. Scientists suspect that scleroderma comes from several factors that may include:

- **Abnormal immune or inflammatory activity:** Like many other rheumatic disorders, scleroderma is believed to be an autoimmune disease. An autoimmune disease is one in which the immune system, for unknown reasons, turns against one's own body.

- **Genetic makeup:** Although genes seem to put certain people at risk for scleroderma and play a role in its course, the disease is not passed from parent to child like some genetic diseases.

- **Environmental triggers:** Researchers suspect that exposure to some environmental factors may trigger scleroderma.

- **Hormones:** Women develop most types of scleroderma more often than men. Scientists suspect that hormonal differences between women and men might play a part in the disease.

Who Gets Scleroderma?

Although scleroderma is more common in women, the disease also occurs in men and children. It affects people of all races and ethnic groups. However, there are some patterns by disease type. For example:

- **Localized forms** of scleroderma are more common in people of European descent than in African Americans. Morphea usually appears between the ages of 20 and 40, and linear scleroderma usually occurs in children or teenagers.

- **Systemic scleroderma,** whether limited or diffuse, typically occurs in people from 30 to 50 years old. It affects more women of African American than European descent.

Because scleroderma can be hard to diagnose and it overlaps with or resembles other diseases, scientists can only estimate how many cases there actually are. It is estimated that 49,000 adults in the United States have systemic sclerosis.

For some people, scleroderma (particularly the localized forms) is fairly mild and resolves with time. But for others, living with the disease and its effects day to day has a significant impact on their quality of life.

How Is Scleroderma Diagnosed?

Depending on your particular symptoms, a diagnosis of scleroderma may be made by:

- A **general internist.**

- A **dermatologist,** who specializes in treating diseases of the skin, hair, and nails.

- An **orthopaedist,** who treats bone and joint disorders.

- A **pulmonologist,** who is trained to treat lung problems.

- A **rheumatologist,** who specializes in treating musculoskeletal disorders and rheumatic diseases.

A diagnosis of scleroderma is based largely on the medical history and findings from the physical exam, questions about what has happened to you over time, and about any symptoms you may be experiencing. Once your doctor has taken a thorough medical history, he or she will perform a physical exam, which can help the doctor diagnose a certain form of scleroderma.

Finally, your doctor may order lab tests to help confirm a suspected diagnosis. The presence of certain antibodies is common in people with scleroderma, but having these antibodies does not confirm the presence of the disease.

In some cases, your doctor may order a skin biopsy (the surgical removal of a small sample of skin for microscopic examination) to aid in or help confirm a diagnosis. However, skin biopsies also have their limitations: biopsy results cannot distinguish between localized and systemic disease, for example.

Diagnosing scleroderma is easiest when a person has typical symptoms and rapid skin thickening. In other cases, a diagnosis may take months, or even years, as the disease unfolds and reveals itself and as the doctor is able to rule out some other potential causes of the symptoms.

How Is Scleroderma Treated?

Because scleroderma can affect many different organs and organ systems, you may have several different doctors involved in your care. Typically, care will be managed by a rheumatologist (a doctor specializing in treatment of musculoskeletal disorders and rheumatic diseases). Your rheumatologist may refer you to other specialists, depending on the specific problems you are having. For example, you may see a dermatologist for the treatment of skin symptoms, a nephrologist for kidney complications, a cardiologist for heart complications, a gastroenterologist for problems of the digestive tract, and a pulmonary specialist for lung involvement.

In addition to doctors, professionals such as nurse practitioners, physician assistants, physical or occupational therapists, psychologists, and social workers may play a role in your care. Dentists, orthodontists, and even speech therapists can treat oral complications that arise from thickening of tissues in and around the mouth and on the face.

Currently, there is no treatment that controls or stops the underlying problem—the overproduction of collagen—in all forms of scleroderma. Thus, treatment and management focus on relieving symptoms and limiting damage. Your treatment will depend on the particular problems you are having. Some treatments will be prescribed or given by your doctor. Others are things you can do on your own.

Stiff, painful joints: In diffuse systemic sclerosis, hand joints can stiffen because of hardened skin around the joints or inflammation within them. Other joints can also become stiff and swollen.

- Stretching exercises under the direction of a physical or occupational therapist are extremely important to prevent loss of joint motion.

- Exercise regularly. Ask your doctor or physical therapist about an exercise plan that will help you increase and maintain range of motion in affected joints.

- Use medication as recommended by your doctor to help relieve joint or muscle pain. If pain is severe, speak to a rheumatologist about the possibility of prescription-strength drugs to ease pain and inflammation.

- Learn to do things in a new way. A physical or occupational therapist can help you learn to perform daily tasks, such as lifting and carrying objects or opening doors, in ways that will put less stress on tender joints.

Skin problems: When too much collagen builds up in the skin, it crowds out sweat and oil glands, causing the skin to become dry and stiff. If your skin is affected, try the following:

- Apply oil-based creams and lotions frequently, and always right after bathing.

- Apply sunscreen before you venture outdoors to protect against further damage from the sun's rays.

- Use humidifiers to moisten the air in your home in colder winter climates. Clean humidifiers often to stop bacteria from growing in the water.

- Avoid very hot baths and showers, as hot water dries the skin.

- Avoid harsh soaps, household cleaners, and caustic chemicals, if at all possible. Otherwise, be sure to wear rubber gloves when you use such products.

- Exercise regularly. Exercise, especially swimming, stimulates blood circulation to affected areas.

Dry mouth and dental problems: Dental problems are common in people with scleroderma for a number of reasons:

- Tightening facial skin can make the mouth opening smaller and narrower, which makes it hard to care for teeth.

- Dry mouth caused by salivary gland damage speeds up tooth decay.

- Damage to connective tissues in the mouth can lead to loose teeth.

You can avoid tooth and gum problems in several ways:

- Brush and floss your teeth regularly. If hand pain and stiffness make this difficult, consult your doctor or an occupational therapist about specially made toothbrush handles and devices to make flossing easier.

- Have regular dental checkups. Contact your dentist immediately if you experience mouth sores, mouth pain, or loose teeth.

- If decay is a problem, ask your dentist about fluoride rinses or prescription toothpastes that remineralize and harden tooth enamel.

- Consult a physical therapist about facial exercises to help keep your mouth and face more flexible.

- Keep your mouth moist by drinking plenty of water, sucking ice chips, using sugarless gum and hard candy, and avoiding mouthwashes with alcohol. If dry mouth still bothers you, ask your doctor about a saliva substitute or medications that can stimulate the flow of saliva.

Gastrointestinal (GI) problems: Systemic sclerosis can affect any part of the digestive system. As a result, you may experience problems such as heartburn, difficulty swallowing, early satiety (the feeling of being full after you've barely started eating), or intestinal complaints such as diarrhea, constipation, and gas. In cases where the intestines are damaged, your body may have difficulty absorbing nutrients from food. Although GI problems are diverse, here are some things that might help at least some of the problems you have:

- Eat small, frequent meals.

- To keep stomach contents from backing up into the esophagus, stand or sit for at least an hour (preferably 2 or 3 hours) after eating.

- When it is time to sleep, keep the head of your bed raised using blocks.

- Avoid late-night meals, spicy or fatty foods, alcohol, and caffeine, which can aggravate GI distress.

- Eat moist, soft foods, and chew them well. If you have difficulty swallowing or if your body doesn't absorb nutrients properly, your doctor may prescribe a special diet.

- Ask your doctor about medications for problems such as diarrhea, constipation, and heartburn. Some drugs called proton pump inhibitors are highly effective against heartburn. Oral antibiotics may stop bacterial overgrowth in the bowel, which can be a cause of diarrhea in some people with systemic sclerosis.

Lung damage: Virtually all people with systemic sclerosis have some loss of lung function. Some develop severe lung disease, which comes in two forms; pulmonary fibrosis (hardening or scarring of lung tissue because of excess collagen) and pulmonary hypertension (high blood pressure in the artery that carries blood from the heart to the lungs). Treatment for the two conditions is different:

- Pulmonary fibrosis may be treated with drugs that suppress the immune system, along with low doses of corticosteroids.

- Pulmonary hypertension may be treated with drugs that dilate the blood vessels or with newer medications that are prescribed specifically for treating pulmonary hypertension.

Regardless of your particular lung problem or its medical treatment, your role in the treatment process is essentially the same. To minimize lung complications, work closely with your medical team. Do the following:

- Watch for signs of lung disease, including fatigue, shortness of breath or difficulty breathing, and swollen feet. Report these symptoms to your doctor.

- Have your lungs closely checked, using standard lung-function tests, during the early stages of skin thickening. These tests, which can find problems at the earliest and most treatable stages, are needed because lung damage can occur even before you notice any symptoms.

- Get regular flu and pneumonia vaccines as recommended by your doctor. Contracting either illness could be dangerous for a person with lung disease.

Heart problems: Common among people with scleroderma, heart problems include scarring and weakening of the heart (cardiomyopathy), inflamed heart muscle (myocarditis), and abnormal heartbeat (arrhythmia). All of these problems can be treated. Treatment ranges from drugs to surgery and varies depending on the nature of the condition.

Kidney problems: Renal crisis is an uncommon but serious complication in patients with systemic sclerosis. Renal crisis results in severe uncontrolled high blood pressure, which can quickly lead to kidney failure. It's very important that you take measures to identify and treat the hypertension as soon as it occurs. These are things you can do:

- Check your blood pressure regularly. You should also check it if you have any new or different symptoms such as a headache or shortness of breath. If your blood pressure is higher than usual, call your doctor right away.

- If you have kidney problems, take your prescribed medications faithfully. In the past two decades, drugs known as ACE (angiotensin-converting enzyme) inhibitors have made scleroderma-related kidney failure a less threatening problem than it used to be. But for these drugs to work, you must take them as soon as the hypertension is present.

Cosmetic problems: Even if scleroderma doesn't cause any lasting physical disability, its effects on the skin's appearance—particularly on the face—can take their toll on your self-esteem. Fortunately, there are procedures to correct some of the cosmetic problems scleroderma causes:

- The appearance of telangiectasias—small red spots on the hands and face caused by swelling of tiny blood vessels beneath the skin—may be reduced or even eliminated with the use of guided lasers.

- Facial changes of localized scleroderma—such as the *en coup de sabre* that may run down the forehead in people with linear scleroderma—may be corrected through cosmetic surgery. (However, such surgery is not appropriate for areas of the skin where the disease is active.)

Chapter 38

Urticaria (Hives)

What Is Urticaria?

Urticaria, commonly known as hives, is a condition in which itchy, swollen red wheals or welts of different sizes appear on the skin. Although there are many possible causes of hives, they most commonly result from an allergic reaction to food or drugs. Hives can last from several minutes to several hours, or in some cases several weeks. They can be itchy, painful, and sometimes cause a burning sensation. Hives may form in one small area on the surface of the skin, or on a larger area of the body. They affect one out of every five people at some point in life.

There are two distinct types of urticaria, acute and chronic. Acute urticaria typically lasts for less than six weeks. The rashes appear suddenly and disappear within a short period of time. Chronic hives, on the other hand, last for more than six weeks and sometimes for months. Although the condition is not dangerous, it can cause considerable discomfort. Angioedema is another form of hives in which the swelling occurs beneath the surface of the skin, often around the eyes and lips.

Hives are generally not life threatening and do not have long-term health effects. However, when breathing difficulties, dizziness, and swelling of the throat or tongue occur along with an eruption of hives on the skin, it could signal anaphylaxis—a severe, life-threatening allergic reaction—and emergency medical care must be sought.

Causes And Treatment

Hives usually occur as a symptom of allergic reactions, when the body's immune system releases histamines and other chemicals into the bloodstream. Hives may be triggered by contact with a variety of common allergens, including foods, drugs, latex, pollen, insect bites, or dust mites. Urticaria may also occur as a result of bacterial and viral infections; immunizations; disease conditions such as vasculitis and lupus; adverse reactions to blood transfusions; or skin contact with plants such as poison ivy. In some cases, hives may also be caused by external triggers such as exercise, emotional stress, heat and cold, and sun exposure.

While the cause of hives may be obvious in people with known allergies, other people may need to undergo medical testing by specialists to identify the cause. In some people with chronic hives, the underlying cause may be difficult to find. It may be helpful to keep a diary of symptoms, noting the conditions under which they occur and improve. This information can help people identify and avoid any factors that can trigger the condition.

As the first course of treatment for hives, a healthcare provider will usually prescribe antihistamine medication to negate the effects of histamines released into the bloodstream. Corticosteroids may be prescribed if the symptoms are severe. If the patient experiences hives as part of a severe allergic reaction and has symptoms of anaphylaxis, they will require an immediate shot of epinephrine. Anti-itch medications or salves may also be prescribed to provide relief from itching. Applying wet compresses or taking a cool bath with baking soda or oatmeal sprinkled in the water can also help relieve symptoms of hives.

References

1. Cole, Gary W. "Hives (Urticaria and Angiodema)." MedicineNet, n.d.

2. "Hives (Urticaria)," American College of Allergy, Asthma, and Immunology, 2014.

3. "Hives," Medline Plus, September 8, 2014.

Chapter 39

Vitiligo

What Is Vitiligo?

Vitiligo is a pigmentation disorder in which melanocytes (the cells that make pigment) in the skin are destroyed. As a result, white patches appear on the skin in different parts of the body. Similar patches also appear on both the mucous membranes (tissues that line the inside of the mouth and nose) and the retina (inner layer of the eyeball). The hair that grows on areas affected by vitiligo sometimes turns white.

The cause of vitiligo is not known, but doctors and researchers have several different theories. There is strong evidence that people with vitiligo inherit genes that make them susceptible to depigmentation. The most widely accepted view is that the depigmentation occurs because vitiligo is an autoimmune disease—a disease in which a person's immune system reacts against the body's own organs or tissues. People's bodies produce proteins called cytokines that, in vitiligo, alter their pigment-producing cells and cause these cells to die. Another theory is that melanocytes destroy themselves. Finally, some people have reported that a single event, such as sunburn or emotional distress, triggered vitiligo; however, these events have not been scientifically proven as causes of vitiligo.

Who Is Affected By Vitiligo?

About 0.5 to 1 percent of the world's population have vitiligo. The average age of onset is in the mid-twenties, but it can appear at any age. The disorder affects both sexes and all races equally; however, it is more noticeable in people with dark skin.

About This Chapter: This chapter includes text excerpted from "Vitiligo—Questions And Answers About Vitiligo," National Institute of Arthritis and Musculoskeletal and Skin Diseases (NIAMS), October 2016.

Vitiligo seems to be somewhat more common in people with certain autoimmune diseases, including hyperthyroidism (an overactive thyroid gland), adrenocortical insufficiency (the adrenal gland does not produce enough of the hormone called corticosteroid), alopecia areata (patches of baldness), and pernicious anemia (a low level of red blood cells caused by the failure of the body to absorb vitamin B12). Scientists do not know the reason for the association between vitiligo and these autoimmune diseases. However, most people with vitiligo have no other autoimmune disease.

Vitiligo sometimes runs in families. Children whose parents have the disorder are more likely to develop vitiligo. However, most children will not get vitiligo even if a parent has it, and most people with vitiligo do not have a family history of the disorder.

What Are The Symptoms Of Vitiligo?

People who develop vitiligo usually first notice white patches (depigmentation) on their skin. These patches are more commonly found on sun-exposed areas of the body, including the hands, feet, arms, face, and lips. Other common areas for white patches to appear are the armpits and groin and around the mouth, eyes, nostrils, navel, genitals, and rectum.

Vitiligo generally appears in one of two patterns:

- **Segmental (or unilateral) pattern**—depigmented patches that develop on one side of the body only.

- **Nonsegmental (or bilateral or generalized) pattern**—the most common pattern. Depigmentation occurs symmetrically on both sides of the body.

In addition to white patches on the skin, people with vitiligo may have premature graying of the scalp hair, eyelashes, eyebrows, and beard. People with dark skin may notice a loss of color inside their mouths.

Will The Depigmented Patches Spread?

Segmental vitiligo remains localized to one part of the body and does not spread. There is no way to predict if nonsegmental vitiligo will spread. For some people, the depigmented patches do not spread. The disorder is usually progressive, however, and over time the white patches will spread to other areas of the body. For some people, vitiligo spreads slowly, over many years. For other people, spreading occurs rapidly. Some people have reported additional depigmentation following periods of physical or emotional stress.

How Is Vitiligo Diagnosed?

The diagnosis of vitiligo is made based on a physical examination, medical history, and laboratory tests.

A doctor will likely suspect vitiligo if you report (or the physical examination reveals) white patches of skin on the body, particularly on sun-exposed areas, including the hands, feet, arms, face, and lips. If vitiligo is suspected, the doctor will ask about your medical history. Important factors in the diagnosis include a family history of vitiligo; a rash, sunburn, or other skin trauma that occurred at the site of vitiligo before depigmentation started; stress or physical illness; and premature graying of the hair (usually before age 35). In addition, the doctor will ask whether you or anyone in your family has had any autoimmune diseases and whether you are very sensitive to the sun.

To help confirm the diagnosis, the doctor may take a small sample (biopsy) of the affected skin to examine under a microscope. In vitiligo, the skin sample will usually show a complete absence of pigment-producing melanocytes. On the other hand, the presence of inflamed cells in the sample may suggest that another condition is responsible for the loss of pigmentation.

Because vitiligo may be associated with pernicious anemia (a condition in which an insufficient amount of vitamin B12 is absorbed from the gastrointestinal tract) or hyperthyroidism (an overactive thyroid gland), the doctor may also take a blood sample to check the blood cell count and thyroid function. For some patients, the doctor may recommend an eye examination to check for uveitis (inflammation of part of the eye), which sometimes occurs with vitiligo. A blood test to look for the presence of antinuclear antibodies (a type of autoantibody) may also be done. This test helps determine if the patient has another autoimmune disease.

How Can People Cope With The Emotional And Psychological Aspects Of Vitiligo?

Although vitiligo is usually not harmful medically, it's emotional and psychological effects can be devastating.

White patches of vitiligo can affect emotional and psychological well-being and self-esteem. People with vitiligo can experience emotional stress, particularly if the condition develops on visible areas of the body (such as the face, hands, arms, and feet) or on the genitals. Adolescents, who are often particularly concerned about their appearance, can be devastated by widespread vitiligo. Some people who have vitiligo feel embarrassed, ashamed, depressed, or worried about how others will react.

Fortunately, there are several strategies to help people cope with vitiligo. Also, various treatments—discussed in the next section—can minimize, camouflage, or, in some cases, even eliminate white patches. First, it is important to find a doctor who is knowledgeable about the disorder and takes it seriously. You must let your doctor know if you are feeling depressed, because doctors and other mental health professionals can help people deal with depression. You should also learn as much as possible about the disorder and treatment choices so that you can participate in making important decisions about your medical care.

What Treatment Options Are Available?

The main goal of treating vitiligo is to reduce the contrast in color between affected and unaffected skin. The choice of therapy depends on the number of white patches; their location, sizes, and how widespread they are; and what you prefer in terms of treatment. Each patient responds differently to therapy, and a particular treatment may not work for everyone. Current treatment options for vitiligo include medication, surgery, and adjunctive therapies (used along with surgical or medical treatments).

Medical Therapies

A number of medical therapies, most of which are applied topically, can reduce the appearance of vitiligo. These are some of the most commonly used:

- **Topical therapy.** Creams, including corticosteroids, may be helpful in repigmenting (returning the color to) white patches, particularly if they are applied in the initial stages of the disease. Corticosteroids are a group of drugs similar to hormones such as cortisone, which are produced by the adrenal glands. Yet, as with any medication, these creams can cause side effects. For this reason, the doctor will monitor you closely for skin shrinkage and skin striae (streaks or lines on the skin).

- **Light treatment.** Light therapy or excimer laser treatments are also used to treat vitiligo, although multiple treatments are needed and results may not be permanent.

- **Psoralen photochemotherapy.** Also known as psoralen and ultraviolet A (PUVA) therapy, this is an effective treatment for many patients. The goal of PUVA therapy is to repigment the white patches. However, it is time consuming, and care must be taken to avoid side effects, which can sometimes be severe. Psoralen is a drug that contains chemicals that react with ultraviolet light to cause darkening of the skin. The treatment involves taking psoralen by mouth (orally) or applying it to the skin (topically). This is followed by carefully timed exposure to sunlight or to ultraviolet A (UVA) light that comes from a special lamp. You must minimize exposure to sunlight at other times.

Known side effects of oral psoralen include sunburn, nausea and vomiting, itching, abnormal hair growth, and hyperpigmentation. Oral psoralen photochemotherapy may also increase the risk of skin cancer, although the risk is minimal at doses used for vitiligo. If you are undergoing oral PUVA therapy, you will be advised to apply sunscreen, avoid direct sunlight, and wear protective UVA sunglasses for a period of time after each treatment.

- **Depigmentation.** This treatment involves fading the rest of the skin on the body to match the areas that are already white. For people who have vitiligo on more than 50 percent of their bodies, depigmentation may be recommended. Patients apply cream once or twice a day to pigmented areas until they match the already depigmented areas. The major side effect of depigmentation therapy is inflammation (redness and swelling) of the skin. You may also experience itching or dry skin. Depigmentation tends to be permanent, is time consuming, and is not easily reversed. In addition, a person who undergoes depigmentation will always be unusually sensitive to sunlight.

Surgical Therapies

Surgical techniques may be an option when topical creams and light therapy do not work. Surgery is typically not recommended for people who scar easily or develop keloids. A variety of effective procedures are available. Talk to your doctor about whether a surgical approach may be right for you.

Additional Therapies

In addition to medical and surgical therapies, there are many things you can do on your own to protect your skin, minimize the appearance of white patches, and cope with the emotional aspects of vitiligo:

- **Sunscreens.** People who have vitiligo, particularly those with fair skin, should minimize sun exposure and use a sunscreen that provides protection from both UVA and ultraviolet B light. Tanning makes the contrast between normal and depigmented skin more noticeable. Sunscreen helps protect the skin from sunburn and long-term damage.

- **Cosmetics.** Some patients with vitiligo cover depigmented patches with makeup, self-tanning lotions or dyes. These cosmetic products can be particularly effective for people whose vitiligo is limited to exposed areas of the body.

- **Counseling and support groups.** Many people with vitiligo find it helpful to get counseling from a mental health professional. People often find they can talk to a counselor about issues that are difficult to discuss with anyone else. A mental health counselor can also offer support and help in coping with vitiligo. In addition, it may be helpful to attend a vitiligo support group.

Part Five
Skin Injuries

Chapter 40

Scrapes, Cuts, And Bruises

Wounds are injuries that break the skin or other body tissues. They include cuts, scrapes, scratches, and punctured skin. They often happen because of an accident, but surgery, sutures, and stitches also cause wounds. Minor wounds usually aren't serious, but it is important to clean them. Serious and infected wounds may require first aid followed by a visit to your doctor. You should also seek attention if the wound is deep, you cannot close it yourself, you cannot stop the bleeding or get the dirt out, or it does not heal.

You Can Injure Your Skin

It's not too hard to injure your skin. So be careful when you're doing anything that might injure it (like using sharp tools, working in the yard, or playing a sport). Cuts, bumps, and scrapes are a normal part of life. It wouldn't be much fun if you tried to avoid them completely. But it's smart to wear the right protective equipment, like gloves, long sleeves, knee and elbow pads, or helmets.

Be very careful when you're around anything hot that can burn your skin. Burns, including sunburn, can be very painful and can take a long time to heal. Burns can also get infected easily.

About This Chapter: Text in this chapter begins with excerpts from "Wounds And Injuries," MedlinePlus, National Institutes of Health (NIH), July 23, 2014; Text under the heading "You Can Injure Your Skin" is excerpted from "Healthy Skin Matters," National Institute of Arthritis and Musculoskeletal and Skin Diseases (NIAMS), October 2015; Text under the heading "How To Care For Minor Wounds" is excerpted from "Emergency Wound Care After A Natural Disaster," Centers for Disease Control and Prevention (CDC), June 20, 2014; Text under the heading "Treating Deep Cuts And Lacerations" is excerpted from "Safety, Health, And Environmental Training—First Aid Basics," U.S. Department of Agriculture (USDA), August 12, 2016; Text under the heading "Bruises" is © 2018 Omnigraphics. Reviewed August 2017.

Sometimes, burns leave bad scars and permanently damage your skin. If you're helping out in the kitchen, make sure you use hot pads or wear oven mitts to protect your hands when you're grabbing something hot.

If you do get a cut or scratch, clean it right away with soap and warm water and put on a bandage to protect it while it heals. This keeps dirt and germs from getting into the wound and causing an infection. If you come into contact with a plant like poison ivy, wash your skin and clothing right away. If you develop a rash, ask your pharmacist about over-the-counter medicines. For severe rashes, you might need to see your doctor.

How To Care For Minor Wounds

- Wash your hands thoroughly with soap and clean water if possible.

- Avoid touching the wound with your fingers while treating it (if possible, use disposable, latex gloves).

- Remove obstructive jewelry and clothing from the injured body part.

- Apply direct pressure to any bleeding wound to control bleeding.

- Clean the wound after bleeding has stopped.

  - Examine wounds for dirt and foreign objects.

  - Gently flood the wound with bottled water or clean running water (if available, saline solution is preferred).

  - Gently clean around the wound with soap and clean water.

  - Pat dry and apply an adhesive bandage or dry clean cloth.

- Leave unclean wounds, bites, and punctures open. Wounds that are not cleaned correctly can trap bacteria and result in infection.

- Provide pain relievers when possible.

Seek medical attention as soon as possible if:

- There is a foreign object (soil, wood, metal, or other objects) embedded in the wound;

- The wound is at special risk of infection (such as a dog bite or a puncture by a dirty object);

- An old wound shows signs of becoming infected (increased pain and soreness, swelling, redness, draining, or you develop a fever).

Other considerations:

- Expect a variety of infection types from wounds exposed to standing water, sea life, and ocean water.

- Wounds in contact with soil and sand can become infected.

- Puncture wounds can carry bits of clothing and dirt into wounds and result in infection.

- Crush injuries are more likely to become infected than wounds from cuts.

- Take steps to prevent tetanus.

What Is First Aid?

First aid refers to medical attention that is usually administered immediately after the injury occurs and at the location where it occurred. It often consists of a one-time, short-term treatment and requires little technology or training to administer. First aid can include:

- cleaning minor cuts, scrapes, or scratches;
- treating a minor burn;
- applying bandages and dressings;
- the use of nonprescription medicine;
- draining blisters;
- removing debris from the eyes;
- massage;
- drinking fluids to relieve heat stress.

(Source: "Medical And First Aid," Occupational Safety and Health Administration (OSHA).)

Treating Deep Cuts And Lacerations

It is very important for you to get immediate treatment for every injury, regardless how small you may think it is. Many cases have been reported where a small unimportant injury, such as a splinter wound or a puncture wound, quickly led to an infection, threatening the health and limb of the employee. Even the smallest scratch is large enough for dangerous germs to enter, and in large bruises or deep cuts, germs come in by the millions.

Control Bleeding With Pressure

Bleeding is the most visible result of an injury. Each of us has between five and six quarts of blood in our body. Most people can lose a small amount of blood with no problem, but if a quart or more is quickly lost, it could lead to shock and/or death.

- One of the best ways to treat bleeding is to place a clean cloth on the wound and apply pressure with the palm of your hand until the bleeding stops.

- Elevate the wound above the victim's heart, if possible, to slow down the bleeding at the wound site.

- Apply pressure to the nearest supplying blood vessel (major pressure point) located either on the inside of the upper arm between the shoulder and elbow, or in the groin area where the leg joins the body.

Direct pressure is better than a pressure point or a tourniquet because direct pressure stops blood circulation only at the wound.

Once the bleeding stops, do not try to remove the cloth that is against the open wound as it could disturb the blood clotting and restart the bleeding. Only use the pressure points if elevation and direct pressure haven't controlled the bleeding.

Never use a tourniquet (a device, such as a bandage twisted tight with a stick, to control the flow of blood) except in response to an extreme emergency, such as a severed arm or leg. Tourniquets can damage nerves and blood vessels and can cause the victim to lose an arm or leg.

Bruises

Produced by blunt trauma to the muscle, a muscle contusion or bruise is second only to strain as the leading type of injury that occurs in sports. A contusion can result from a simple fall or from the impact of jamming the body against a hard surface. Contusions do not involve a break in the skin. However, injury occurs to the soft tissues, including muscle fiber, blood vessels, or nerves. The injury typically shows up as a discoloration (ecchymoses) on the skin and is characterized by pain, tenderness, and swelling. The discoloration, caused by the pooling of blood from a ruptured blood vessel, starts off as a reddish-purple mark and changes color to blue-black, and eventually greenish-yellow as healing progresses. Muscle contusions are most common in contact sports such as football, boxing, and rugby.

Grading Of Muscle Contusions: Like sprains, contusions are graded depending on the severity:

- **Mild:** Caused by rupture of a small blood vessel, this is the least severe of contusions and is mostly asymptomatic. There is little or no pain and minimal loss of muscle function, and the individual can immediately return to his or her sport or activity.

- **Moderate:** Injury is slightly deeper than a mild contusion and involves pain, swelling, and a moderate loss of movement around the site of injury. Healing and return to activity after this type of injury usually takes anywhere between three and four weeks.

- **Severe:** This results from a massive blunt force to deep muscle tissues and is typically characterized by the formation of an intramuscular hematoma (a blood clot formed from a massive rupture of a blood vessel). When touched, the hematoma can be felt as a firm lump. This type of contusion is almost always accompanied by inflammation, intense pain, and complete loss of muscle function.

Treatment

As with any type of soft tissue injury, the first line therapy for muscle contusion is the RICE (rest, ice, compression, and elevation) regimen. This treatment should be administered as soon as possible after the injury to reduce hemorrhage (bleeding), muscle spasms, and inflammation.

Depending on the site and extent of injury, the elements of RICE therapy may be used together or as a combination of two or more elements.

- **Rest:** Conservative treatment of muscle contusion begins with immobilization of the injury site. A short period of early immobilization not only helps speedy repair of muscle tissues but also prevents chances of re-injury.

- **Ice:** The use of ice (also called cryotherapy) is effective in managing the acute phase (24–48 hours after injury) of a muscle contusion. Ice helps to reduce hemorrhage and thereby decreases the size of the hematoma. This, in turn, lowers inflammation and speeds up the regeneration of muscle tissue. Ice is usually applied for no longer than 15–20 minutes at a time.

- **Compression:** Wrapping the injured area with a bandage helps to reduce bleeding and edema (fluid buildup). Care should be taken to ensure a snug-fitting bandage. However, a wrapping that is too tight will cut off adequate blood flow to the injured muscle and cause more harm than good.

- **Elevation:** Raising the injured area to or above the level of your heart also helps to reduce pain and swelling by draining the excess fluid around the injured tissue back to the body's circulatory system.

Chapter 41

Scars And Scar Removal

What Is A Scar?

A scar is the result of the skin repairing itself from injury. It is a pale pink, brown, or silvery patch of skin that grows where you had a cut, scrap, or other injury. People get hurt all the time and scars are a part of life. Any kind of injury—such as burns, cuts, serious trauma, or surgery—can result in a scar. Many scars are small and easy to conceal, but if a scar is large, in a prominent place, or just makes you feel self-conscious, you may wish to remove it. If so, several methods exist to reduce the size and minimize the appearance of scars, but removing a scar completely is nearly impossible.

How Is A Scar Formed?

When skin is injured, it produces collagen—tough fibers of protein that are white in color—which reconnects the broken tissue like bridges. As the wound heals, a scab, which is a dry crust made of blood platelets and other substances, forms over the wound. The scab protects the wound as it heals. Over time, the scab falls away leaving behind repaired skin and more often a scar.

What Are The Types Of Scars?

Scars are classified into the following types:

- **Keloid scars.** A keloid scar is a raised, thick, and irregular patch of tissue that forms beyond the margins of the original wound. They are also darker in color when compared

"Scars And Scar Removal," © 2018 Omnigraphics. Reviewed August 2017.

to surrounding tissue. Unlike other scars, keloid scars do not regress over time, and can, in fact, continue to grow. They commonly occur in the chest, back, shoulders, and earlobes. Researchers believe that keloid scars are the result of an overactive healing process.

- **Hypertrophic scars.** Hypertrophic scars are raised, pale-colored scars that do not expand beyond the area of injury. The scar tissue is thicker than the surrounding tissue.

- **Contracture scars.** These scars occur when tissue is lost due to injury. During the healing process, the edges of the skin pull together and tighten, possibly impairing movement. Severe burns often result in contracture scars.

- **Acne scars.** This common skin condition can result in deep, pitted scars.

How Should You Care For Wounds To Reduce Scarring?

The chance that a wound can result in a scar has a lot to do with how the wound is treated. If you do get hurt:

- Get wounds treated immediately.

- Cover the wound in a way that keeps infection out but allows a scab to form.

- Avoid picking at the scab, which can increase the likelihood of scarring.

- If recommended by your doctor, use special bandages silicone sheets to keep pressure on the wound. This will flatten any resulting scarring.

Once the wound has healed, you can minimize any resulting scar by massaging the area to help break the dense collagen forming in the tissue. Also, if a scar becomes inflamed, red, or itchy, it may be infected and should be treated by a medical professional.

What Are The Treatment Options For Scars?

Doctors have a range of procedures and treatments available to them to help reduce the size and appearance of scars. They include:

- **Cryosurgery.** Cryosurgery is used to freeze the upper layers of the scar, causing them to blister and slough off. This treatment option is primarily used for keloids.

- **Punch grafts.** Used to treat acne scars, this procedure takes healthy skin, usually from the earlobes, and grafts it onto small holes punched in the scarred region.

- **Chemical peels.** A chemical is applied to the skin and removed, removing a thin layer of cells from the top of the skin. Chemical peels are used to treat sun-damaged and lightly scarred skin.

- **Cortisone injections.** Intralesional steroid injections are used to soften and shrink hard scars, including keloid and hypertrophic scars.

- **Dermabrasion.** Top layers of the skin are abraded using an electrical machine. As the skin surface heals, the skin will appear smoother and more even. This is used to treat acne scars.

- **Surgical scar revision.** The scar is surgically removed and the skin is rejoined, creating a new, less prominent scar. Surgical scar revision is usually done to treat scars that are very wide and visible on the patient's body.

- **Laser resurfacing.** A laser beam is used to destroy the top layer of skin, resulting in a new layer that appears smoother and more even. This treatment is generally used to treat hypertrophic scars.

- **Silicone dioxide.** This chemical is applied in gel or pad form to reduce the redness of keloids.

- **Pressure therapy.** Keloids are treated by wearing a pressure appliance over the scar for 4—6 months.

References

1. "The Story On Scars," The Nemours Foundation, February 2015.

2. Gardner, Stephanie S., MD. "Cosmetic Procedures: Scars," WebMD, LLC, January 18, 2016.

3. "Scars," American Society for Dermatologic Surgery (ASDS), n.d.

4. Berman, Kevin, MD, PhD, Sather, Rita, RN. "Scars," University of Rochester Medical Center Rochester, 2017.

Chapter 42

Burn Injuries

What Is A Burn?

A burn is tissue damage caused by heat, chemicals, electricity, sunlight, or nuclear radiation. The most common burns are those caused by scalds, building fires, and flammable liquids and gases.

- First-degree burns affect only the outer layer (the epidermis) of the skin.

- Second-degree burns damage the epidermis and the layer beneath it (the dermis).

- Third-degree burns involve damage or complete destruction of the skin to its full depth and damage to underlying tissues.

Every day, over 300 children ages 0 to 19 are treated in emergency rooms for burn-related injuries and two children die as a result of being burned.

Younger children are more likely to sustain injuries from scald burns that are caused by hot liquids or steam, while older children are more likely to sustain injuries from flame burns that are caused by direct contact with fire.

(Source: "Protect The Ones You Love: Child Injuries Are Preventable—Burn Prevention," Centers for Disease Control and Prevention (CDC).)

About This Chapter: This chapter includes text excerpted from "Burns Fact Sheet," National Institute of General Medical Sciences (NIGMS), November 2012. Reviewed August 2017.

How Does The Body React To A Severe Burn?

The swelling and blistering characteristic of burns is caused by the loss of fluid from damaged blood vessels. In severe cases, such fluid loss can cause shock. Burns often lead to infection, due to damage to the skin's protective barrier.

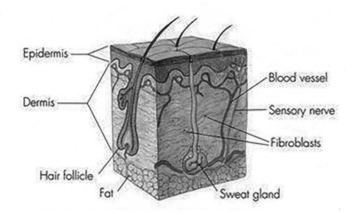

Figure 42.1. Skin

How Are Burns Treated?

In many cases, topical antibiotics (skin creams or ointments) are used to prevent infection. For third-degree burns and some second-degree one's, immediate blood transfusion and/or extra fluids are needed to maintain blood pressure. Grafting with natural or artificial materials speeds the postburn healing process.

First Aid For Burns

For minor burns:

- Immerse in fresh, cool water,
- or apply cool compresses for 10-15 minutes.
- Dry the area with a clean cloth. Cover with sterile gauze or a nonadhesive bandage.
- Don't apply ointments or butter; these may cause infection.
- Don't break blisters.
- Over-the-counter pain medications may help reduce inflammation and pain.

Call emergency services (911) if:

- burns cover a large area of the body.
- burns affect the entire thickness of skin.
- the victim is an infant or elderly.
- the burn was caused by electricity, which can lead to "invisible" burns.

(Source: "A Burning Issue," NIH News in Health, National Institutes of Health (NIH).)

What Is Skin Grafting?

There are two types of skin grafts. An autologous skin graft transfers skin from one part of the body to another while an allograft transfers skin from another person, sometimes even a cadaver. Scientists typically take cells from the epidermal layer of skin and then grow them into large sheets of cells in the laboratory. They do not yet know how to grow the lower, dermal layer of skin in the lab. For this reason, surgeons, after removing burned skin, first cover the area with an artificial material and then add the cell sheets on top. This procedure helps encourage the growth of new skin.

What Is The Prognosis For Severe Burn Victims?

A few decades ago, burns covering half the body were often fatal. Now, thanks to research, many people with burns covering 90 percent of their bodies can survive, although they often have permanent impairments and scars.

Where Are People Treated For Burns?

Over half of burn patients in the United States are treated in specialized burn centers, and most hospitals have trauma teams that care exclusively for patients with traumatic injuries that may accompany burns.

How Has Basic Research Improved Burn Care?

Remarkable improvements in burn care have resulted from basic research funded by the National Institutes of Health (NIH). The results have led to the best approaches for fluid resuscitation, wound cleaning, skin replacement, infection control and nutritional support.

What Is On The Horizon For Burn Research?

Improving methods for wound healing and tissue repair offer tremendous opportunities to enhance the quality of life for burn patients and may also help to reduce healthcare costs.

Chapter 43

What You Should Know About Animal Bites

Animal Bites

Wild animals usually avoid people. They might attack, however, if they feel threatened, are sick, or are protecting their young or territory. Attacks by pets are more common. Animal bites rarely are life-threatening, but if they become infected, you can develop serious medical problems.

To prevent animal bites and complications from bites:

- Never pet, handle, or feed unknown animals

- Leave snakes alone

- Watch your children closely around animals

- Vaccinate your cats, ferrets, and dogs against rabies

- Spay or neuter your dog to make it less aggressive

- Get a tetanus booster if you have not had one recently

- Wear boots and long pants when you are in areas with venomous snakes

If an animal bites you, clean the wound with soap and water as soon as possible. Get medical attention if necessary.

About This Chapter: Text under the heading "Animal Bites" is excerpted from "Animal Bites," MedlinePlus, National Institutes of Health (NIH), January 5, 2015; Text under the heading "Snake Bite" is excerpted from "How To Prevent Or Respond To A Snake Bite," Centers for Disease Control and Prevention (CDC), June 20, 2014; Text under the heading "Dog Bite" is excerpted from "Healthy Pets Healthy People—Dogs," Centers for Disease Control and Prevention (CDC), July 14, 2016; Text under the heading "Catscratch Disease" is excerpted from "Cat-Scratch Disease (CSD)," Centers for Disease Control and Prevention (CDC), April 30, 2014.

Snake Bite

Highlights

- If you see a snake in your home, immediately call the animal control agency in your county.

- Be aware of snakes that may be swimming in the water or hiding under debris or other objects.

- If you or someone you know are bitten, try to see and remember the color and shape of the snake.

- Do not pick up a snake or try to trap it.

After a natural disaster, snakes may have been forced from their natural habitats and move into areas where they would not normally be seen or expected. When you return to your home, be cautious of snakes that may have sought shelter in your home.

How To Prevent Snake Bites

- Be aware of snakes that may be swimming in the water to get to higher ground and those that may be hiding under debris or other objects.

- If you see a snake, back away from it slowly and do not touch it.

Signs Of Snake Bites

If you have to walk in high water, you may feel a bite, but not know that you were bitten by a snake. You may think it is another kind of bite or scratch. Pay attention to the following snake bite signs. Depending on the type of snake, the signs and symptoms may include:

- A pair of puncture marks at the wound
- Redness and swelling around the bite
- Severe pain at the site of the bite
- Nausea and vomiting
- Labored breathing (in extreme cases, breathing may stop altogether)
- Disturbed vision
- Increased salivation and sweating
- Numbness or tingling around your face and/or limbs

What TO DO If You Or Someone Else Is Bitten By A Snake

- If you or someone you know are bitten, try to see and remember the color and shape of the snake, which can help with treatment of the snake bite.

- Keep the bitten person still and calm. This can slow down the spread of venom if the snake is poisonous.

- Seek medical attention as soon as possible.

- Dial 911 or call local Emergency Medical Services (EMS).

- Apply first aid if you cannot get the person to the hospital right away.

  - Lay or sit the person down with the bite below the level of the heart.

  - Tell him/her to stay calm and still.

  - Cover the bite with a clean, dry dressing.

What NOT TO DO If You Or Someone Else Is Bitten By A Snake

- Do not pick up the snake or try to trap it (this may put you or someone else at risk for a bite).

- Do not apply a tourniquet.

- Do not slash the wound with a knife.

- Do not suck out the venom.

- Do not apply ice or immerse the wound in water.

- Do not drink alcohol as a pain killer.

- Do not drink caffeinated beverages.

Dog Bite

Many studies show the health benefits of dog ownership. Dogs not only provide comfort and companionship, but several studies have found that dogs decrease stress and promote relaxation. Dogs have positive impacts on nearly all life stages. They influence social, emotional, and cognitive development in children, promote an active lifestyle, and have even been able to detect oncoming epileptic seizures or the presence of certain cancers. But for all the positive benefits of keeping dogs, pet owners should be aware that dogs can carry germs that make people sick.

Although germs from dogs rarely spread to people, they might cause a variety of illnesses, ranging from minor skin infections to serious disease. To protect yourself and your family from getting sick:

- Seek routine veterinary care for your pet and

- Always wash your hands and the hands of children with running water and soap after contact with dogs, their stool, and their food.

By providing your pet with routine veterinary care and some simple health tips, you are less likely to get sick from touching, petting, or owning dogs in the United States.

Diseases

The most common diseases associated with dogs that can cause human illness are:

Campylobacteriosis (*Campylobacter* spp.)

Campylobacter spreads through contaminated food (meat and eggs), water, or contact with stool of infected animals. Dogs infected with *Campylobacter* might show no signs of illness at all or might have diarrhea and a slight fever.

Most people who become sick with campylobacteriosis will have diarrhea, cramping, abdominal pain, and fever within 2–5 days after exposure to the organism. *Campylobacter* can cause serious life-threatening infections in infants, older persons, and those with weakened immune systems.

Dog Tapeworm (*Dipylidium caninum*)

The dog tapeworm is a parasite spread to dogs, cats, and people through the ingestion of infected fleas. This parasite is common but rarely causes illness in pets or people. Infections with *Dipylidium caninum* can sometimes be detected by finding rice-like segments of the tapeworm crawling near the anus or in fresh bowel movements. In severe infections, pets can lose weight and have mild diarrhea.

In people, children are more commonly infected but don't usually show signs of disease. The best way to prevent infection in pets is to control the flea population in the environment.

Hookworm (Zoonotic) (*Ancylostoma caninum, Ancylostoma braziliense, Uncinaria stenocephala*)

Dog hookworms are tiny worms that can spread through contact with contaminated soil or sand. Dogs can also become infected with hookworms through accidentally ingesting the parasite from the environment or through their mother's milk or colostrum. Young puppies are most often affected and might have dark, bloody stool and anemia. Severe infections in some puppies can lead to death.

People become infected with dog hookworms while walking barefoot, kneeling, or sitting on ground contaminated with stool of infected animals. Hookworm larvae enter the top layers of skin and cause an itchy reaction called cutaneous larva migrans. A red squiggly line might appear where the larvae have migrated under the skin. Symptoms usually resolve without medical treatment in 4–6 weeks.

Rabies

Rabies, a fatal neurologic disease in animals and people, is caused by a virus. Animals and people are most commonly infected through bites from rabid animals. Infected dogs might have a variety of signs, but most often have a sudden behavioral change and progressive paralysis. Rabies is prevented by vaccination.

The first symptoms in people can start days to months after exposure and include generalized weakness, fever, and headache. Within a few days symptoms will progress to confusion, anxiety, behavioral changes, and delirium. If you have been bitten by a dog or other animal and feel that there is a risk for rabies, contact your healthcare provider right away. Once symptoms appear, it is almost always too late for treatment.

Roundworm (*Toxocara* spp.)

Toxocara roundworms cause a parasitic disease known as toxocariasis. Dogs and people can become infected by accidentally swallowing roundworm eggs from the environment. In addition, larval worms can cross through the placenta, milk, or colostrum of a mother dog, passing the infection to her puppies. Infected puppies usually do not develop and grow well and might have a pot-bellied appearance.

In people, children are most often affected with roundworm. There are two forms of the disease in people. Ocular larva migrans happens when the larvae invade the retina and cause inflammation, scarring, and possibly blindness. Visceral larva migrans occurs when the larvae invade parts of the body, such as the liver, lung, or central nervous system.

Preventing Dog Bites

About 4.5 million Americans receive dog bites each year, many of which require immediate medical attention. Young children 5 to 9 years old are most likely to bitten by dogs, with boys being bitten more often than girls.

What To Do If You Are Bitten Or Scratched By A Dog

Germs can be spread from dog bites and scratches, even if the wound does not seem deep or serious. If a bite from a dog occurs, you should—

- Wash wounds with warm soapy water immediately.

- Seek medical attention:

    - If you don't know if the dog has been vaccinated against rabies

    - If the dog appears sick or is acting strangely

    - If the wound is serious (uncontrolled bleeding, loss of function, extreme pain, muscle or bone exposure, etc.)

    - If the wound becomes red, painful, warm or swollen, or if you develop a fever

    - If it has been more than 5 years since your last tetanus shot

    - If you have any concerns about your or your child's health

- Report the bite to your local animal control or health department.

    - If possible, contact the owner and ensure the animal has a current rabies vaccination. You will need the rabies vaccine license number, name of the veterinarian that administered the vaccine, and the owner's name, address, and phone number.

- Due to the risk of rabies, ensure that the dog is seen by a veterinarian and contact your local health department if it becomes sick or dies within 10 days of the bite.

Catscratch Disease

Catscratch disease (CSD) is a bacterial infection spread by cats. The disease spreads when an infected cat licks a person's open wound, or bites or scratches a person hard enough to break the surface of the skin. About three to 14 days after the skin is broken, a mild infection can occur at the site of the scratch or bite. The infected area may appear swollen and red with round, raised lesions and can have pus. The infection can feel warm or painful. A person with CSD may also have a fever, headache, poor appetite, and exhaustion. Later, the person's lymph nodes closest to the original scratch or bite can become swollen, tender, or painful.

Wash cat bites and scratches well with soap and running water. Do not allow cats to lick your wounds. **Contact your doctor** if you develop any symptoms of catscratch disease or infection.

CSD is caused by a bacterium called *Bartonella henselae.* About 40 percent of cats carry B. henselae at some time in their lives, although most cats with this infection show NO signs of illness. Kittens younger than 1 year are more likely to have *B. henselae* infection and to spread the germ to people. Kittens are also more likely to scratch and bite while they play and learn how to attack prey.

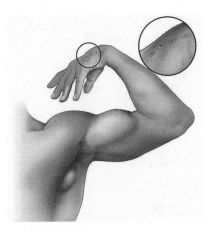

Figure 43.1. Catscratch Disease (CSD)

An enlarged lymph node in the armpit region of a person with catscratch disease, and wounds from a cat scratch on the hand.

How Cats And People Become Infected

Cats can get infected with *B. henselae* from flea bites and flea dirt (droppings) getting into their wounds. By scratching and biting at the fleas, cats pick up the infected flea dirt under their nails and between their teeth. Cats can also become infected by fighting with other cats that are infected. The germ spreads to people when infected cats bite or scratch a person hard enough to break their skin. The germ can also spread when infected cats lick at wounds or scabs that you may have.

Serious But Rare Complications

People

Although rare, CSD can cause people to have serious complications. CSD can affect the brain, eyes, heart, or other internal organs. These rare complications, which may require intensive treatment, are more likely to occur in children younger than 5 years and people with weakened immune systems.

Cats

Most cats with *B. henselae* infection show NO signs of illness, but on rare occasions this disease can cause inflammation of the heart—making cats very sick with labored breathing. *B. henselae* infection may also develop in the mouth, urinary system, or eyes. Your veterinarian may find that some of your cat's other organs may be inflamed.

Prevention

People

Do:

- Wash cat bites and scratches right away with soap and running water.
- Wash your hands with soap and running water after playing with your cat, especially if you live with young children or people with weakened immune systems.
- Since cats less than one year of age are more likely to have CSD and spread it to people, persons with a weakened immune system should adopt cats older than one year of age.

Do not:

- Play rough with your pets because they may scratch and bite.
- Allow cats to lick your open wounds.
- Pet or touch stray or feral cats.

Cats

Control Fleas

- Keep your cat's nails trimmed.
- Apply a flea product (topical or oral medication) approved by your veterinarian once a month.
  - **BEWARE:** Over-the-counter flea products may not be safe for cats. Check with your veterinarian before applying ANY flea product to make sure it is safe for your cat and your family.
- Check for fleas by using a flea comb on your cat to inspect for flea dirt.
- Control fleas in your home by:
  - Vacuuming frequently
  - Contacting a pest-control agent if necessary

Protect Your Cat's Health

- Schedule routine veterinary health check-ups.
- Keep cats indoors to:
  - Decrease their contact with fleas
  - Prevent them from fighting with stray or potentially infected animals

Available Tests And Treatments

People

Talk to your doctor about testing and treatments for CSD. People are only tested for CSD when the disease is severe and the doctor suspects CSD based on the patient's symptoms. CSD is typically not treated in otherwise healthy people.

Cats

Talk to your veterinarian about testing and treatments for your cat. Your veterinarian can tell you whether your cat requires testing or treatment.

Chapter 44

Insect Bites And Stings

Warm weather makes it easier to spend more time outdoors, but it also brings out the bugs. Ticks are usually harmless. But a tick bite can lead to Lyme disease, which is caused by the bacterium *Borrelia burgdorferi*. The bacteria are transmitted to people by the black-legged deer tick, which is about the size of a pinhead and usually lives on deer. Infected ticks can also cause other diseases, such as Rocky Mountain spotted fever.

Another insect-borne illness, West Nile virus, is transmitted by infected mosquitoes and usually produces mild symptoms in healthy people. But the illness can be serious for older people and those with compromised immune systems.

Most reactions to bees and other stinging insects are mild, but severe allergic reactions can be deadly. An allergic reaction can occur even if a person has been stung before with no complications.

What Can I Do To Keep Insects Away?

Here are tips for preventing and treating bites and stings.

- Use structural barriers such as window screens and netting.

- Avoid wooded, brushy, and grassy areas when possible.

- Don't wear heavily scented soaps and perfumes.

- Use caution eating outside and drinking; don't leave drinks and garbage cans uncovered.

About This Chapter: This chapter includes text excerpted from "Beware Of Bug Bites And Stings," U.S. Food and Drug Administration (FDA), October 3, 2016.

- Don't wear bright colors, which attract bees.

- Wear long sleeves and long pants when possible.

- Tuck pant legs into socks or shoes.

- Wear a hat for extra protection.

- Get rid of containers with standing water that give mosquitoes a breeding ground. Examples include water in flowerpots and outdoor pet dishes.

- Use insect repellent if nonchemical methods are ineffective and you spend time in tall grass and woody areas.

- Treat camping gear, clothes, and shoes with permethrin, which repels and kills ticks, mosquitoes, and other insects. Clothing that is pretreated with permethrin is also commercially available.

What's The Proper Way To Use Insect Repellent?

It's okay to use insect repellent and sunscreen at the same time. The general recommendation is to apply sunscreen first, followed by repellent. There are also some combination products that contain both insect repellent and sunscreen. U.S. Food and Drug Administration (FDA) regulates sunscreen as an over-the-counter (OTC) drug. The Environmental Protection Agency (EPA) regulates insect repellent products.

- Use insect repellent that contains active ingredients that have been registered with EPA. An EPA registration number on the product label means the product has been evaluated by EPA to ensure that it will not pose unreasonable harmful effects on people and the environment.

- Spray insect repellent on clothes or skin, but not on the face.

- Don't use insect repellent on babies. Repellent used on older children should contain no more than 10 percent DEET. Oil of eucalyptus products should not be used in children under 3 years.

- Don't use insect repellent that's meant for people on your pets.

- Use insect repellent according to the labeled instructions.

- Avoid applying it to children's hands, around the eyes, or to areas where there are cuts and irritated skin.

- Store insect repellent out of children's reach.

- Wash the repellent off with soap and water and contact a Poison Control Center (800-222-1222) if you (or your child) experience a reaction to insect repellent.

- After returning indoors, wash skin with soap and water to remove repellent.

What's The Best Way To Remove A Bee Stinger?

It's best to scrape a stinger away in a side-to-side motion with a straight-edged object like a credit card. Don't use tweezers because it may push more venom into the skin. After removing a stinger, wash the area with soap and water. You can apply ice or another cold compress to help reduce swelling.

What Should I Do If I Find A Tick On Me Or My Child?

Wearing light-colored clothing makes it easier to spot ticks. Check for ticks after outdoor activities. If you find a tick, remove it with tweezers. Grasp the tick as close to the skin as possible and pull it straight out. Then drop it in a plastic bag, seal it up, and throw it away. Early removal of a tick is important because a tick generally has to be on the skin for 36 hours to transmit Lyme disease. People who want to get a tick tested for disease or other information could check with their local health departments to see if they offer tick testing. After removing a tick, you can cleanse the area of the tick bite with antiseptic, such as rubbing alcohol or soap and water.

What Can Be Done For Itching And Pain From Bites And Stings?

Oral OTC antihistamines can bring itch relief. Oral OTC drugs, such as ibuprofen and acetaminophen, can provide relief of pain from bites and stings.

In addition, there are many topical OTC drugs that are applied to the skin and can provide itch and pain relief. Some of these topical OTC drugs are labeled as "external analgesics" or "topical analgesics." They contain ingredients such as hydrocortisone, pramoxine, and lidocaine. There are also topical OTC drugs labeled as "skin protectants" that provide itch relief for insect bites and stings. These products contain ingredients such as colloidal oatmeal and sodium bicarbonate.

Keep kids' nails short. If they scratch the area and break the skin, it can lead to a bacterial infection that will require treatment with antibiotics.

When Is Medical Attention Needed?

Most bites and stings are minor and can be treated at home. But you should seek medical attention if you experience the following symptoms:

- **Signs of allergic reaction:** Some people can experience anaphylaxis, a severe, life-threatening allergic reaction. This is a medical emergency that warrants calling 9-1-1 immediately. Signs of an allergic reaction, which may occur within seconds to minutes, include sneezing, wheezing, hives, nausea, vomiting, diarrhea, sudden anxiety, dizziness, difficulty breathing, chest tightness, and itching or swelling of the eyes, lips, or other areas of the face. If you or your child has ever had an allergic reaction to a sting or bite, you should be evaluated by an allergist. In some cases, you may be advised to wear a medical identification tag that states the allergy, and to carry epinephrine, a medication used to treat serious or life-threatening allergic reactions. Sometimes allergy shots may also be recommended.

- **Symptoms of Lyme disease:** Lyme disease, which is transmitted through the bite of an infected tick, can cause fever, headaches, fatigue, and a skin rash that looks like a circular red patch, or "bull's-eye." Left untreated, infection can spread to the joints, heart, and nervous system. It is rarely, if ever, fatal. Patients who are treated with antibiotics in the early stages of the infection usually recover rapidly and completely. Antibiotics commonly used for oral treatment include doxycycline, amoxicillin, or cefuroxime axetil (Ceftin). People with certain illnesses related to the heart or the nervous system require intravenous treatment with drugs such as ceftriaxone or penicillin.

- **Symptoms of West Nile virus:** West Nile virus, which is transmitted by infected mosquitoes, can produce flu-like symptoms including fever, headache, body aches, and skin rash. While most infected individuals have mild disease and recover spontaneously, infection can be serious or even fatal. There is no specific treatment for West Nile virus.

- **Symptoms of Rocky Mountain spotted fever:** Initial symptoms may include fever, nausea, vomiting, severe headache, muscle pain, and lack of appetite. The characteristic red, spotted rash of Rocky Mountain spotted fever is usually not seen until the sixth day or later after symptoms begin. But as many as 10 percent to 15 percent of patients may never develop a rash. Rocky Mountain spotted fever is treated with antibiotics.

- **Signs of infection:** It is normal for a bite or sting to result in redness of the affected area and minor swelling. But if a bite or sting becomes infected, a fever may develop or the redness or soreness may worsen. In cases of infection, an antibiotic is the typical treatment.

Chapter 45

Protecting Yourself From Poisonous Plants

Many native and exotic plants are poisonous to humans when ingested or if there is skin contact with plant chemicals. However, the most common problems with poisonous plants arise from contact with the sap oil of several native plants that cause an allergic skin reaction— poison ivy, poison oak, and poison sumac.

Recognizing Poison Ivy, Poison Oak, And Poison Sumac

- **Poison Ivy:** Found throughout the United States except Alaska, Hawaii, and parts of the West Coast. Can grow as a vine or small shrub trailing along the ground or climbing on low plants, trees and poles. Each leaf has three glossy leaflets, with smooth or toothed edges. Leaves are reddish in spring, green in summer, and yellow, orange, or red in fall. May have greenish-white flowers and whitish-yellow berries.

- **Poison Oak:** Grows as a low shrub in the Eastern and Southern United States, and in tall clumps or long vines on the Pacific Coast. Fuzzy green leaves in clusters of three are lobed or deeply toothed with rounded tips. May have yellow-white berries.

- **Poison Sumac:** Grows as a tall shrub or small tree in bogs or swamps in the Northeast, Midwest, and parts of the Southeast. Each leaf has clusters of seven to 13 smooth-edged leaflets. Leaves are orange in spring, green in summer, and yellow, orange, or red in fall. May have yellow-greenish flowers and whitish-green fruits hang in loose clusters.

(Source: "Outsmarting Poison Ivy And Other Poisonous Plants," U.S. Food and Drug Administration (FDA).)

About This Chapter: Text in this chapter begins with excerpts from "Poisonous Plants," National Institute for Occupational Safety and Health (NIOSH), Centers for Disease Control and Prevention (CDC), July 7, 2016; Text beginning with the heading "Symptoms Of Skin Contact" is excerpted from "NIOSH Fast Facts: Protecting Yourself From Poisonous Plants," National Institute for Occupational Safety and Health (NIOSH), Centers for Disease Control and Prevention (CDC), June 6, 2014.

Outdoor workers may be exposed to poisonous plants. Outdoor workers at risk include farmers, foresters, landscapers, groundskeepers, gardeners, painters, roofers, pavers, construction workers, laborers, mechanics, and any other workers who spend time outside. Forestry workers and firefighters who battle forest fires are at additional risk because they could potentially develop rashes and lung irritation from contact with damaged or burning poisonous plants.

Symptoms Of Skin Contact

- Red rash within a few days of contact

- Swelling

- Itching

- Possible bumps, patches, streaking, or weeping blisters

Poison Plant Rashes Aren't Contagious

Poison ivy and other poison plant rashes can't be spread from person to person. But it is possible to pick up the rash from plant oil that may have stuck to clothing, pets, garden tools, and other items that have come in contact with these plants. The plant oil lingers (sometimes for years) on virtually any surface until it's washed off with water or rubbing alcohol.

(Source: "Outsmarting Poison Ivy And Other Poisonous Plants," U.S. Food and Drug Administration (FDA).)

First Aid

If you are exposed to a poisonous plant:

- Immediately rinse skin with rubbing alcohol, poison plant wash, or degreasing soap (such as dishwashing soap) or detergent, and lots of water.

  - Rinse frequently so that wash solutions do not dry on the skin and further spread the urushiol.

- Scrub under nails with a brush.

- Apply wet compresses, calamine lotion, or hydrocortisone cream to the skin to reduce itching and blistering.

  - Oatmeal baths may relieve itching.

- An antihistamine may help relieve itching.

  - NOTE: Drowsiness may occur.

- In severe cases or if the rash is on the face or genitals, seek professional medical attention.

- Call 911 or go to a hospital emergency room if you have a severe allergic reaction, such as swelling or difficulty breathing, or have had a severe reaction in the past.

Protect Yourself

- Wear long sleeves, long pants, boots, and gloves.

  - Wash exposed clothing separately in hot water with detergent.

- Barrier skin creams, such as lotion containing bentoquatum, may offer some protection.

- After use, clean tools with rubbing alcohol or soap and lots of water. Urushiol can remain active on the surface of objects for up to 5 years.

  - Wear disposable gloves during this process.

- Do not burn plants or brush piles that may contain poison ivy, poison oak, or poison sumac.

  - Inhaling smoke from burning plants can cause severe allergic respiratory problems.

Chapter 46

Frostbite

Frostbite is a serious condition that's caused by exposure to extremely cold temperatures. Stay safe this winter by learning more about frostbite, including who is most at risk, signs and symptoms, and what to do if someone develops frostbite.

What Is Frostbite?

Frostbite is a bodily injury caused by freezing that results in loss of feeling and color in affected areas. It most often affects the nose, ears, cheeks, chin, fingers, or toes. Frostbite can permanently damage the body, and severe cases can lead to amputation.

Who's Most At Risk?

You may have a greater risk of developing frostbite if you:

- Have poor blood circulation

- Are not properly dressed for extremely cold temperatures

Recognizing Frostbite

At the first signs of redness or pain in any skin area, get out of the cold or protect any exposed skin—frostbite may be beginning. Any of the following signs may indicate frostbite:

- a white or grayish-yellow skin area

About This Chapter: Text in this chapter begins with excerpts from "Frostbite," Centers for Disease Control and Prevention (CDC), December 20, 2016; Text under the heading "Frostbite Caution" is excerpted from "Frostbite Caution," Centers for Disease Control and Prevention (CDC), October 25, 2016.

- skin that feels unusually firm or waxy

- numbness

A victim is often unaware of frostbite until someone else points it out because the frozen tissues are numb.

What To Do

If you detect symptoms of frostbite, seek medical care. First, determine whether the victim also shows signs of hypothermia. Hypothermia is a more serious medical condition and requires emergency medical assistance.

If (1) there is frostbite but no sign of hypothermia and (2) immediate medical care is not available, proceed as follows:

- Get into a warm room as soon as possible.

- Unless absolutely necessary, do not walk on frostbitten feet or toes—this increases the damage.

- Immerse the affected area in warm—not hot—water (the temperature should be comfortable to the touch for unaffected parts of the body).

- Or, warm the affected area using body heat. For example, the heat of an armpit can be used to warm frostbitten fingers.

- Do not rub the frostbitten area with snow or massage it at all. This can cause more damage.

- Don't use a heating pad, heat lamp, or the heat of a stove, fireplace, or radiator for warming. Affected areas are numb and can be easily burned.

These procedures are not substitutes for proper medical care. Hypothermia is a medical emergency and frostbite should be evaluated by a healthcare provider.

Be Prepared

Taking a first aid and emergency resuscitation (CPR) course is a good way to prepare for cold-weather health problems. Knowing what to do is an important part of protecting your health and the health of others.

Taking preventive action is your best defense against having to deal with extreme cold-weather conditions. By preparing your home and car in advance for winter emergencies, and by observing safety precautions during times of extremely cold weather, you can reduce the risk of weather-related health problems.

Frostbite Caution

Since skin may be numb, victims of frostbite can harm themselves further.

Use caution when treating frostbite and:

1. Unless necessary, do not walk on feet or toes with frostbite

2. Do not use a fireplace, heat lamp, radiator, or stove for warming

3. Do not use a heating pad or electric blanket for warming

4. Do not rub or massage areas with frostbite

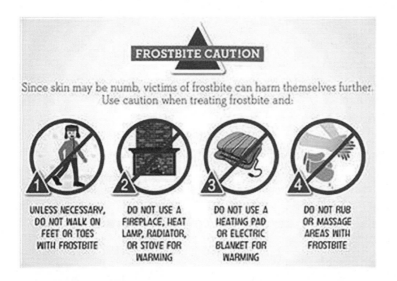

Figure 46.1. Frostbite Caution

Chapter 47

Blisters, Corns, And Calluses

About Blisters

Blisters are fluid-filled sacs on the outer layer of your skin. They form because of rubbing, heat, or diseases of the skin. They are most common on your hands and feet.

Other names for blisters are vesicles (usually for smaller blisters) and bulla (for larger blisters).

Causes Of Blisters

Blisters often happen when there is friction—rubbing or pressure—on one spot. For example, if your shoes don't fit quite right and they keep rubbing part of your foot. Or if you don't wear gloves when you rake leaves and the handle keeps rubbing against your hand. Other causes of blisters include:

- Burns

- Sunburn

- Frostbite

- Eczema

- Allergic reactions

About This Chapter: Text beginning with the heading "About Blisters" is excerpted from "Blisters," MedlinePlus, National Institutes of Health (NIH), November 15, 2016; Text beginning with the heading "About Corns And Calluses" is excerpted from "Corns And Calluses," National Institutes of Health (NIH), August 25, 2016; Text beginning with the heading "Taking Care Of Your Feet Is Important" is excerpted from "Be Sweet To Your Feet," *NIH News in Health,* National Institutes of Health (NIH), September 2016.

- Poison ivy, oak, and sumac
- Autoimmune diseases such as pemphigus
- Epidermolysis bullosa, an illness that causes the skin to be fragile
- Viral infections such as varicella zoster (which causes chickenpox and shingles) and herpes simplex (which causes cold sores)
- Skin infections including impetigo

Treatments For Blisters

Blisters will usually heal on their own. The skin over the blister helps keep out infections. You can put a bandage on the blister to keep it clean. Make sure that there is no more rubbing or friction on the blister.

You should contact your healthcare provider if:

- The blister looks infected—if it is draining pus, or the area around the blister is red, swollen, warm, or very painful
- You have a fever
- You have several blisters, especially if you cannot figure out what is causing them
- You have health problems such as circulation problems or diabetes

Normally you don't want to drain a blister, because of the risk of infection. But if a blister is large, painful, or looks like it will pop on its own, you can drain the fluid.

Things To Do To Prevent Blisters

There are some things you can do to prevent friction blisters:

- Make sure that your shoes fit properly
- Always wear socks with your shoes, and make sure that the socks fit well. You may want to wear socks that are acrylic or nylon, so they keep moisture away from your feet.
- Wear gloves or protective gear on your hands when you use any tools or sports equipment that cause friction.

About Corns And Calluses

Corns and calluses are caused by pressure or friction on your skin. They often appear on feet where the bony parts of your feet rub against your shoes. Corns usually appear on the tops or sides of toes while calluses form on the soles of feet. Calluses also can appear on hands or other areas that are rubbed or pressed.

Wearing shoes that fit better or using nonmedicated pads may help. While bathing, gently rub the corn or callus with a washcloth or pumice stone to help reduce the size. To avoid infection, do not try to shave off the corn or callus. See your doctor, especially if you have diabetes or circulation problems.

Smooth Corns And Calluses Gently

If you have corns or calluses, talk with your foot doctor about the best way to care for these foot problems. If you have nerve damage, these patches can become ulcers.

If your doctor tells you to, use a pumice stone to smooth corns and calluses after bathing or showering. A pumice stone is a type of rock used to smooth the skin. Rub gently, only in one direction, to avoid tearing the skin.

Do NOT

- cut corns and calluses

- use corn plasters, which are medicated pads

- use liquid corn and callus removers

Cutting and over-the counter corn removal products can damage your skin and cause an infection.

To keep your skin smooth and soft, rub a thin coat of lotion, cream, or petroleum jelly on the tops and bottoms of your feet. Do not put lotion or cream between your toes because moistness might cause an infection.

Taking Care Of Your Feet Is Important

Your feet work hard to get you where you need to be. But years of wear and tear can be rough on them. So can disease, bad circulation, poorly trimmed toenails, and wearing shoes that don't fit.

So be kind to your feet. Exercise, especially walking, is a great way to increase blood flow, which helps your feet stay healthy. Try simple foot exercises, such as sitting and rotating your ankles one way, then the other.

What To Look For

- Blisters, cuts or scratches can lead to infection if ignored.
- Callus or corns are signs of excessive pressure and need to be addressed immediately.
- Swelling can be a sign of injury to the soft tissue or bone and should be brought to the attention of your footcare specialist immediately.

(Source: "Foot Care For A Lifetime," Health Resources and Services Administration (HRSA).)

Tips For Happy Feet

- Wash your feet regularly, especially between your toes.

- Wear clean socks.

- Wear well-fitting, comfy shoes.

- Wear shoes when you're outside.

- Put your feet up when you're sitting, to help circulation.

- If you're sitting for a long time, stand up and move around every now and then.

- If you cross your legs when sitting, reverse or uncross them often.

Chapter 48

Skin Picking, Nail Biting, And Hair Pulling

Skin picking (excoriation) disorder, nail biting (onychophagia), and hair pulling (trichotillomania) disorder are classified in a set of conditions known as body-focused repetitive behavior (BFRB). They are not habits or tics but self-injurious behavior. These are complex disorders in which people touch themselves repeatedly in ways that cause physical damage.

Skin Picking

Skin picking disorder is a condition in which a person repeatedly touches, picks at, rubs, scratches or digs into skin in an attempt to remove irregularities or perceived imperfections in the skin. The disorder affects as many as 1 in 20 people. It occurs in both men and women but research suggests that it occurs predominantly in women. Exact causes are not known but biological and environmental factors could play a role. The disorder is characterized by people picking at one or more areas of the skin in the body such as the head, face, back, arms, legs, and cuticles.

Skin picking could occur out of boredom or habit and the person is sometimes not aware that it is happening. More often, people use fingers or fingernails to pick their skin but some could bite or use tools like tweezers or scissors. Some people pick their skin as an outlet for negative emotions such as anxiety, sadness, and anger or to deal with stress or mounting tension. Skin picking provides such people with relief but immediately afterwards they undergo feelings of shame and guilt. People dispose of the removed skin in different ways. Some discard it in the trash or on the floor while some people eat it.

About This Chapter: Text in this chapter begins with excerpts from "Skin Picking And Nail Biting," © 2018 Omnigraphics. Reviewed August 2017; Text under the heading "Hair Pulling" is excerpted from "Trichotillomania," Genetic and Rare Diseases Information Center (GARD), National Center for Advancing Translational Sciences (NCATS), August 1, 2017.

Treatment

Skin picking disorder is usually treated with medication and psychological therapy. Understanding why such behavior occurs and finding emotional support goes a long way in addressing the condition. Psychological interventions are also helpful in treating individuals and achieving remission.

Habit reversal training is one form of therapy that is used. During therapy, the healthcare provider helps the patient understand the situations, stressors, and factors that trigger skin picking behavior. The therapist then suggests alternative things the patient can do to relieve the stress such as squeezing a rubber ball. This helps in destressing as well as keeping the hands occupied.

Stimulus control is another form of therapy for treating skin picking disorder. Changes are made to the environment to curb skin picking. A person will be asked to wear gloves or put on Band-Aids to avoid peeling any skin and thus prevent the urge to pick skin. Mirrors are covered so that a person cannot see blemishes on the face or skin and thus avoid skin picking behavior.

Sometimes, psychiatric medications can provide relief but they are not specifically recommended for the condition by the U.S. Department of Food and Drug Administration (FDA). SSRIs (selective serotonin reuptake inhibitors) are a class of psychiatric medications well suited to treat skin picking disorder. The efficacy of anticonvulsants in the treatment of skin picking disorder is currently being researched. Individuals should also consult a dermatologist for skin lesions, wounds, and scars caused due to skin picking disorder.

Nail Biting

The medical term for fingernail biting is "onychophagia." It is a common stress relieving and "nervous habit" in children and adults. People bite nails out of boredom, inactivity, stress, or excitement. Children learn to bite their fingernails from other family members. People bite their nails without being aware of it. They could be on the phone, watching TV, working, or reading and biting their nails at the same time. Nail biting involves biting the nail plate, the tissues in the nail bed, and cuticle as well. Nail biting is related to a host of psychiatric disorders such as obsessive–compulsive disorder (OCD), attention deficit hyperactivity disorder (ADHD), separation anxiety disorder, and oppositional defiant disorder (ODD). It causes physical problems as well. Swallowing of bitten nails can cause stomach infections, fungal infections of the nail plate and surrounding skin, and intestinal parasitic infections. Excessive nail biting can also cause temporomandibular joint pain and dysfunction and dental problems.

Treatment

Treatment measures for nail biting depends on the severity of the condition and could vary between making behavior changes and creating physical barriers to prevent nail biting.

- Nail should be trimmed and filed to avoid biting. This prevents from biting nails and encourages them to keep them attractive.

- Painting nails with bitter tasting polish, the taste of which reminds to stop biting nails.

- Stress management techniques can be used if nail biting is a result of stress or anxiety.

- Substituting another activity for nail biting such as squeezing a ball for distraction.

- Employing a negative physical response to nail biting such as snapping a rubber band worn on a wrist whenever you start to bite your nails serves to change the habit.

References

1. Bhandari, Smitha, MD. "Skin Picking Disorder (Excoriation)," WebMD, LLC, February 24, 2016.

2. "Understanding Skin Picking (Excoriation) Disorder: A Body-Focused Repetitive Behavior," The TLC Foundation for Body-Focused Repetitive Behaviors, n.d.

3. Fama, Jeanne M. Ph.D. "Skin Picking Disorder Fact Sheet," International OCD Foundation (IOCDF), 2010.

4. "Nail-Biting," Healthwise, Inc., October 13, 2016.

5. Wu, Brian, MD. "Onychophagia," New Zealand Dermatological Society, December 2016.

Hair Pulling

Trichotillomania is a disorder characterized by an overwhelming urge to repeatedly pull out one's own hair, resulting in hair loss (alopecia). It is classified under the obsessive-compulsive and related disorders category. Trichotillomania results in highly variable patterns of hair loss. The scalp is the most common area of hair pulling, followed by the eyebrows, eyelashes, pubic and perirectal areas, axillae, limbs, torso, and face. The resulting alopecia can range from thin unnoticeable areas of hair loss to total baldness. Some people chew or swallow the hair they pull out (trichophagy), which can result in gastrointestinal problems or develop a trichobezoar (hairball in the intestines or stomach). In many cases, people with this disorder feel extreme tension when they feel an impulse, followed by relief, gratification or pleasure afterwards. The disorder may be mild and manageable, or severe and debilitating. The cause is unknown, though both environmental and genetic causes have been suspected. Treatment may involve cognitive behavioral therapy, such as habit reversal training (learning to substitute the hair-pulling behavior) and/or drug therapy, but these are not always effective.

Treatment

Behavioral treatment seems to be the most powerful treatment for trichotillomania. Parental involvement is important and should include enough support so that affected children grow well intellectually, physically, and socially. Shaving or clipping hair close to the scalp may be helpful to stop the behavior.

Professional cognitive behavior therapy is recommended if initial approaches are unsuccessful. CBT typically involves self-monitoring (keeping records of the behavior); habit-reversal training; and stimulus control (organizing the environment). CBT is typically effective in highly motivated and compliant patients. The success of therapy may depend on firm understanding of the illness and the cooperation of the family members to help the affected individual comply with treatment. Several courses of CBT may be needed.

No medication has been approved for the treatment of trichotillomania, and medications used have not been consistently effective. Selective serotonin reuptake inhibitors (SSRIs) have been utilized but responses to treatment have not been consistent. Fortunately, several recent studies regarding drug therapy for trichotillomania show promise. While drug therapy alone is currently generally not effective, combination therapy and other treatments may be helpful.

Part Six
Taking Care Of Your Skin, Hair, And Nails

Chapter 49

Skin And Hair Care

Skin Care

Keep It Clean

Washing your skin, especially your hands, is very important for keeping it healthy. Hand washing keeps you from spreading germs to other parts of your body. It also keeps you from spreading germs that could give others a cold or the flu. To help keep your skin from getting dry, use water that's comfortably warm, not too hot, when you take a bath or shower. If your skin is dry or itchy, try a moisturizing cream or lotion.

Enjoy Being In The Sun—But Protect Your Skin

Your skin produces vitamin D when it is exposed to sunshine. Vitamin D helps keep your bones and other body systems healthy. However, too much sun can damage your skin and increase your risk for skin cancer. It may make your skin look old years too soon and can make it less able to fight off infections. Whenever you're outside, use a sunscreen with a sun-protection factor (SPF) of 30 or 45. Apply it evenly, and have a friend or parent help you with the hard-to-reach spots. Follow the directions that tell you how often to reapply it—one application won't last all day!

What About Tanning Beds?

Tanning beds don't offer a safe alternative to natural sunlight. Exposure to ultraviolet (UV) radiation damages your skin, whether the exposure comes from tanning beds or natural

About This Chapter: Text under the heading "Skin Care" is excerpted from "Healthy Skin Matters," National Institute of Arthritis and Musculoskeletal and Skin Diseases (NIAMS), October 2015; Text under the heading "Hair Care" is excerpted from "Looking And Feeling Your Best—Hair Care," girlshealth.gov, Office on Women's Health (OWH), April 15, 2014.

sunlight. This damage increases the risk of skin cancer and premature skin aging just like too much sun. In fact, most tanning beds emit mainly ultraviolet A (UVA) rays, which may increase the risk of melanoma, the deadliest form of skin cancer.

Physical Activity

Being physically active is good for your skin! It increases the flow of blood to the surface of your skin and brings oxygen and nutrients to your whole body. Sweating helps to flush out impurities from your skin. Get 1 hour or more of physical activity every day. This will be good for your skin as well as your heart, lungs, muscles, and other parts of your body. Be sure to drink enough water to replace the fluids you lose when you sweat. If you have any concerns about your health, talk to your doctor or a physical therapist to find out what kinds of activities are right for you.

A Healthy Diet

You really don't need a special diet to keep your skin in good health. Eating a balanced diet will help you maintain a healthy weight and provide a variety of nutrients for your skin and your overall health. A balanced diet:

- Emphasizes fruits, vegetables, whole grains, and fat-free or low-fat dairy products like milk, cheese, and yogurt.

- Includes protein from lean meats, poultry, seafood, beans, eggs, and nuts.

- Is low in solid fats, saturated fats, cholesterol, salt (sodium), added sugars, and refined grains.

- Is as low as possible in trans fats.

- Balances calories taken in through food with calories burned in physical activity to help maintain a healthy weight.

Get Some Sleep

Getting enough sleep helps improve your overall health, which is good for your skin. Teens need at least 9 hours of sleep each night, while adults need about 7 to 9 hours.

See Your Doctor

If you find anything unusual on your skin, like a mole that changes size or color or a patch that looks red or itches, ask a parent or other trusted adult to take a look at it and arrange for you to see a doctor. For skin diseases, it's important to see a doctor as early as possible to prevent permanent damage to your skin.

Start Now

Healthy skin will help you look your best and feel good about how you look. Start healthy habits now while you are young—they will help you keep your skin healthy for the rest of your life.

Hair Care

Short, long, curly, straight, up, down. Hair options can seem endless! Not all of what makes your hair look good comes from the outside, though. Good nutrition, physical activity, staying away from the sun, and other healthy habits can help your hair shine!

Here are some other tips for hair care:

If your hair is oily. Try washing your hair every day. You may also want to try shampoos that are made for oily hair. And stop using hair products that have oil in them, like pomades.

If your hair is dry. You may want to use a moisturizing shampoo made for dry hair. Also use a cream rinse or conditioner. You could also try shampooing less often.

If you see white flakes in your hair or on your shoulders. You most likely have dandruff. Try a dandruff shampoo. If it doesn't help, your doctor may prescribe something stronger.

If you want to dye your hair.

- If possible, you might consider having a professional do this for you.

- If you are dyeing your hair at home, it's best to get someone's help.

- Follow the directions in the package carefully, especially any warnings.

- Do a test before using dye on your hair. Rub a tiny bit of the dye on the inside of your elbow or behind your ear. Leave it there for two days. If you get a rash, don't use the dye on your hair.

- Wear gloves when you apply dye.

- Talk with your doctor if your skin or scalp swells or gets itchy after using any hair product. Even natural products, such as henna dye, can cause an allergic reaction.

If you want to straighten your hair.

- If possible, you might consider having a professional do this for you.

- You can use a relaxer product at home, but it can burn your scalp if you use it the wrong way.

- It's best not to try using a relaxer product by yourself. Get help to make sure you've put it on evenly and you get it all out when you're through.

- Make sure to follow any directions, and don't leave the straightener on too long.

- Keep in mind that straightening your hair can damage it. Try not to straighten it too often. Some hairdressers say around once every two months is okay.

Hair Dyes And Relaxers

Hair dye is used to color your hair. Hair relaxers are used to straighten your hair. Both hair dye and hair relaxers can hurt your skin, hair, and eyes, especially if you are not careful.

Careful and proper use of hair products can help avoid problems and keep you safe from having a reaction. Use the following guidelines when using hair dyes and hair relaxers:

- Follow all directions on the label and in the package.
- Keep hair dyes and relaxers away from your eyes, and do not dye your eyebrows or eyelashes. This can hurt your eyes and may even cause blindness.
- Wear gloves when applying hair dye or relaxers.
- Do not leave the product on longer than the directions say you should. Keep track of time using a clock or a timer.
- Rinse well with water after using hair dye or relaxers.
- Keep hair dyes and relaxers out of the reach of children.
- Do not scratch or brush your scalp for three days before using hair dyes or relaxers.
- Do not dye or relax your hair if your scalp is irritated, sunburned, or damaged.
- Wait at least 14 days after bleaching, relaxing, or perming your hair before using dye.

(Source: "Hair Dyes And Relaxers," U.S. Food and Drug Administration (FDA).)

If you want to make your hair curly.

- If you can, you might consider having a professional do this for you.

- You can use a permanent wave, or "perm" at home, but it's a good idea to get help.

- Make sure to follow any directions, and don't leave it on too long.

If you use hair dryers, curling irons, flat irons, or similar products. Be careful not to over-use them. Dryers and other products that use heat can dry out or break your hair. It's a good idea to take a few days off from time to time.

If you swim in a pool a lot. Protect your hair from chlorine by wearing a swim cap or rinsing out your hair right after swimming. Soaking your hair with regular water before you put on your swim cap can also help.

Chapter 50

Sweating And Preventing Body Odor

What Is Sweating?

Sweat is a clear, salty liquid produced by glands in your skin. Sweating is how your body cools itself. You sweat mainly under your arms and on your feet and palms. When sweat mixes with bacteria on your skin, it can cause a smell.

Sweating a lot is normal when it is hot or when you exercise, are anxious, or have a fever. It also happens during menopause. If you often sweat too much, it's called hyperhidrosis. Causes include thyroid or nervous system disorders, low blood sugar, or another health problem.

All Systems Go

Ever wonder what really happens inside your body to make you sweat? Picture this—when your temperature rises, tiny blood vessels close to your skin open up. This allows your blood to carry the heat in your body away from your hard-working muscles to get closer to the skin. Then, water (sweat) escapes through your sweat glands and onto your skin. When air blows over your wet skin, the sweat evaporates (dries up) and cools your body down. But, on really hot, humid days, there is so much moisture in the air that it can't absorb the sweat from your body. So, to keep your body cool, drink plenty of water, use a fan, or take a dip in the pool.

(Source: "Keeping Your Cool," Centers for Disease Control and Prevention (CDC).)

About This Chapter: Text under the heading "What Is Sweating?" is excerpted from "Sweat," MedlinePlus, National Institutes of Health (NIH), April 2, 2015; Text under the heading "Avoiding Odor" is excerpted from "Sweating," girlshealth.gov, Office on Women's Health (OWH), April 15, 2014; Text under the heading "Risks Of Using Antiperspirants/Deodorants" is excerpted from "Antiperspirants/Deodorants And Breast Cancer," National Cancer Institute (NCI), August 9, 2016.

Sweating too little, anhidrosis, can be life-threatening because your body can overheat. Causes of anhidrosis include dehydration, burns, and some skin and nerve disorders.

Avoiding Odor

Sweat Glands

The average person has about 3 million sweat glands. Sweat glands are classified according to two types: Apocrine glands and eccrine glands. Apocrine glands are specialized sweat glands that can be found only in the armpits and pubic region. These glands secrete a milky sweat that encourages the growth of the bacteria responsible for body odor.

(Source: "Site-Specific Modules—Anatomy—Layers Of The Skin," Surveillance, Epidemiology and End Results Program (SEER), National Cancer Institute (NCI).)

You might think that you are only supposed to sweat when you are hot, but once you hit puberty, you will also sweat when you are nervous. Your sweat glands, which are in places like your armpits, become more active during the teen years. That means you will sweat more, and your sweat will have a smell.

Don't panic! Sweat and smell are normal parts of becoming an adult.

You can follow some simple tips to keep from smelling bad:

- Shower or take a bath every day, making sure to wash your underarms, pubic area, and bottom.

- Use a deodorant, which helps get rid of smells, or an antiperspirant, which decreases sweating, or a product that has both of these in it.

- Talk to your doctor if these things do not work or you are worried about smelling bad.

Risks Of Using Antiperspirants/Deodorants

Because underarm antiperspirants or deodorants are applied near the breast and contain potentially harmful ingredients, several scientists and others have suggested a possible connection between their use and breast cancer. However, no scientific evidence links the use of these products to the development of breast cancer.

Chapter 51

Cosmetics: Tips For Girls

People use cosmetics to enhance their beauty. These products range from lipstick and nail polish to deodorant, perfume, and hairspray. Get the facts before using cosmetics.

General Tips

- Read the label. Follow all directions.

- Wash your hands before you use the product.

- Do not share makeup.

- Keep the containers clean and closed tight when not in use.

- Throw away cosmetics if the color or smell changes.

- Do not use spray cans while you are smoking or near an open flame. It could start a fire.

- Use aerosols or sprays in a place with good air flow.

Eye Make-Up Tips

1. Do not add saliva or water to mascara. You could add germs.

2. Throw away your eye makeup if you get an eye infection.

3. Do not use cosmetics near your eyes unless they are meant for your eyes. For example, do not use lip liner on your eyes.

About This Chapter: Text in this chapter begins with excerpts from "Cosmetics: Tips For Women," U.S. Food And Drug Administration (FDA), October 5, 2016; Text under the heading "FAQs About Cosmetics" is excerpted from "Cosmetics Safety Q&A: Shelf Life," U.S. Food And Drug Administration (FDA), April 21, 2017.

4. Do not dye or tint your eyelashes. U.S. Food And Drug Administration (FDA) has not approved any color additives for permanent dyeing or tinting of your eyelashes or eyebrows.

5. Hold still! Even a slight scratch with the mascara wand or other applicator can result in a serious infection. Do not apply makeup in the car or on the bus.

Bad Reaction To Cosmetics?

FDA does not test cosmetics before they are sold in stores. However, FDA does monitor the safety of cosmetic products. Tell FDA if you have a rash, redness, burns, or other serious problems after using cosmetics.

What Should You Do?

- Stop using the product.

- Call your healthcare provider to find out how to take care of the problem.

Understanding Cosmetic Labels

Read the label including the list of ingredients, warnings, and tips on how to use it safely.

- **Hypoallergenic:** Do not assume that the product will not cause allergic reactions. FDA does not define what it means to be labeled 'hypoallergenic'.

- **Organic or Natural:** The source of the ingredients does not determine how safe it is. Do not assume that these products are safer than products made with ingredients from other sources. FDA does not define what it means to be labeled 'organic' or 'natural'.

- **Expiration Dates:** Cosmetics are not required to have an expiration date. A cosmetic product may go bad if you store it the wrong way like if it is unsealed or in a place that is too warm or too moist.

FAQs About Cosmetics
What Is The Shelf Life Of Cosmetics?

The shelf life for eye-area cosmetics is more limited than for other products. Because of repeated microbial exposure during use by the consumer and the risk of eye infections, some industry experts recommend replacing mascara 3 months after purchase.

Among other cosmetics that are likely to have an unusually short shelf life are certain "all natural" products that may contain plant-derived substances conducive to microbial growth. It also is important for consumers and manufacturers to consider the increased risk of contamination in products that contain nontraditional preservatives, or no preservatives at all.

Consumers should be aware that expiration dates are simply "rules of thumb," and that a product's safety may expire long before the expiration date if the product has not been properly stored. Cosmetics that have been improperly stored—for example, exposed to high temperatures or sunlight, or opened and examined by consumers prior to final sale—may deteriorate substantially before the expiration date. On the other hand, products stored under ideal conditions may be acceptable long after the expiration date has been reached.

What Should I Do If I Have A Reaction (Side Effect) To A Cosmetic Product?

If you have a reaction (side effect) to a cosmetic product, you should:

- tell your doctor or other healthcare provider,
- report it to the cosmetic manufacturer, and
- submit a complaint by reporting the problem to the U.S. Food and Drug Administration (FDA)

What Are "Hypoallergenic" Cosmetics?

Hypoallergenic cosmetics are products that manufacturers claim produce fewer allergic reactions than other cosmetic products. Consumers with hypersensitive skin, and even those with "normal" skin, may be led to believe that these products will be gentler to their skin than nonhypoallergenic cosmetics.

What Precautions Should You Take If You Dye Your Hair?

People who dye their hair should follow these safety precautions:

- Follow the directions in the package. Pay attention to all "Caution" and "Warning" statements.
- Do a patch test before using dye on your hair. Here's how: Rub a tiny bit of the dye on the inside of your elbow or behind your ear. Leave it there for two days. If you get a rash, don't use the dye on your hair. You should do the test each time you dye your hair.

- Never dye your eyebrows or eyelashes. This can hurt your eyes. You might even go blind. FDA does not allow using hair dyes on eyelashes and eyebrows.

- Don't leave the dye on longer than the directions say you should.

- Rinse your scalp well with water after dyeing.

- Wear gloves when you apply the hair dye.

- Never mix different hair dye products. This can hurt your hair and scalp.

What Precautions Should You Take When Using Eye Cosmetics?

If you use eye cosmetics, FDA urges you to follow these safety tips:

- If any eye cosmetic causes irritation, stop using it immediately. If irritation persists, see a doctor.

- Avoid using eye cosmetics if you have an eye infection or the skin around the eye is inflamed. Wait until the area is healed. Discard any eye cosmetics you were using when you got the infection.

- Be aware that there are bacteria on your hands that, if placed in the eye, could cause infections. Wash your hands before applying eye cosmetics.

- Make sure that any instrument you place in the eye area is clean.

- Don't share your cosmetics. Another person's bacteria may be hazardous to you.

- Don't allow cosmetics to become covered with dust or contaminated with dirt or soil. Keep containers clean.

- Don't use old containers of eye cosmetics. Discard mascara three months after purchase.

- Don't store cosmetics at temperatures above 85 degrees F. Cosmetics held for long periods in hot cars, for example, are more susceptible to deterioration of the preservative.

- When applying or removing eye cosmetics, be careful not to scratch the eyeball or other sensitive area. Never apply or remove eye cosmetics in a moving vehicle.

- Don't use any cosmetics near your eyes unless they are intended specifically for that use. For instance, don't use a lip liner as an eye liner. You may be exposing your eyes to contamination from your mouth, or to color additives that are not approved for use in the area of the eye.

- Avoid color additives that are not approved for use in the area of the eye, such as "permanent" eyelash tints and kohl.

Chapter 52

Sun Exposure And Staying Safe

Sunburn is an often painful sign of skin damage from spending too much time outdoors without wearing a protective sunscreen. Years of overexposure to the sun lead to premature wrinkling, aging of the skin, age spots, and an increased risk of skin cancer. In addition to the skin, eyes can get burned from sun exposure. Sunburned eyes become red, dry, and painful, and feel gritty. Chronic exposure of eyes to sunlight may cause pterygium (tissue growth that leads to blindness), cataracts, and perhaps macular degeneration, a leading cause of blindness.

Sunlight exposure is highest during the summer and between 10.00 a.m. and 4.00 p.m. Working outdoors during these times increases the chances of getting sunburned. Snow and light-colored sand reflect ultraviolet (UV) light and increase the risk of sunburn. At work sites with these conditions, UV rays may reach workers' exposed skin from both above and below. Workers are at risk of UV radiation even on cloudy days. Many drugs increase sensitivity to sunlight and the risk of getting sunburn. Some common ones include thiazides, diuretics, tetracycline, doxycycline, sulfa antibiotics, and nonsteroidal anti-inflammatory drugs, such as ibuprofen.

Ultraviolet (UV) rays are a part of sunlight that is an invisible form of radiation. UV rays can penetrate and change the structure of skin cells.

There are three types of UV rays:

1. Ultraviolet A (UVA)

About This Chapter: Text in this chapter begins with excerpts from "Workplace Safety And Health Topics—Sun Exposure," Centers for Disease Control and Prevention (CDC), July 13, 2016; Text under the heading "Tips To Stay Safe In The Sun," is excerpted from "Tips To Stay Safe In The Sun: From Sunscreen To Sunglasses," U.S. Food and Drug Administration (FDA), June 27, 2017.

2. Ultraviolet B (UVB)

3. Ultraviolet C (UVC)

UVA is the most abundant source of solar radiation at the earth's surface and penetrates beyond the top layer of human skin. Scientists believe that UVA radiation can cause damage to connective tissue and increase a person's risk for developing skin cancer. UVB rays penetrate less deeply into skin, but can still cause some forms of skin cancer. Natural UVC rays do not pose a risk to workers because they are absorbed by the Earth's atmosphere.

Symptoms

Unlike a thermal burn, sunburn is not immediately apparent. Symptoms usually start about 4 hours after sun exposure, worsen in 24–36 hours, and resolve in 3–5 days.

Symptoms may include:

- Red, warm, and tender skin
- Swollen skin
- Blistering
- Headache
- Fever
- Nausea
- Fatigue

The pain from sunburn is worse 6–48 hours after sun exposure. Skin peeling usually begins 3–8 days after exposure.

First Aid

There is no quick cure for minor sunburn:

- Symptoms can be treated with aspirin, acetaminophen, or ibuprofen to relieve pain and headache and reduce fever.
- Drinking plenty of water helps to replace fluid losses.
- Cool baths or the gentle application of cool wet cloths on the burned area may also provide some comfort.
- Workers with sunburns should avoid further exposure until the burn has resolved.
- Additional symptomatic relief may be achieved through the application of a topical moisturizing cream, aloe, or 1 percent hydrocortisone cream.

- A low-dose (0.5%–1%) hydrocortisone cream, which is sold over-the-counter, may be helpful in reducing the burning sensation and swelling and speeding up healing.

If blistering occurs:

- Lightly bandage or cover the area with gauze to prevent infection.

- The blisters should not be broken, as this will slow the healing process and increase the risk of infection.

- When the blisters break and the skin peels, dried fragments may be removed and an antiseptic ointment or hydrocortisone cream may be applied.

- Seek medical attention if any of the following occur:

  - Severe sunburns covering more than 15 percent of the body

  - Dehydration

  - High fever (>101°F)

  - Extreme pain that persists for longer than 48 hours

Sun exposure leads to skin cancer such as basal cell, squamous cell, and melanoma.

Some of the symptoms include:

- Irregular borders on moles (ragged, notched, or blurred edges).

- Moles that are not symmetrical (one half doesn't match the other).

- Colors that are not uniform throughout.

- Moles that are bigger than a pencil eraser.

- Sores that bleed and do not heal.

- Itchy or painful moles.

- Red patches or lumps.

- New moles.

Tips To Stay Safe In The Sun

Sun safety is always in season, and it's important to protect your skin from sun damage throughout the year, no matter the weather. Why? Exposure to the sun can cause sunburn, skin aging (such as skin spots, wrinkles, or "leathery skin"), eye damage, and skin cancer, the most common of all cancers.

And skin cancer is on the rise in the United States. The Centers for Disease Control and Prevention (CDC) estimates there were more than 71,943 people diagnosed with melanoma of the skin—the most serious form of skin cancer—in 2013 alone. About 4.3 million people are treated for basal cell cancer and squamous cell skin cancer in the United States every year, according to a 2014 report from the Office of the Surgeon General.

The U.S. Food and Drug Administration (FDA) is continuing to evaluate sunscreen products to ensure available sunscreens help protect consumers from sunburn. If products claim to help protect from skin cancer and early skin aging caused by the sun, the FDA also evaluates these products to ensure they help protect consumers from these issues when used as directed with other sun protection measures.

Reduce Your Risk For Sunburn, Skin Cancer, And Early Skin Aging Caused By The Sun

Sun damage to the body is caused by invisible ultraviolet (UV) radiation. Sunburn is a type of skin damage caused by the sun. Tanning is also a sign of the skin reacting to potentially damaging UV radiation by producing additional pigmentation that provides it with some—but often not enough—protection against sunburn.

Spending time in the sun increases your risk of skin cancer and early skin aging. People of all skin colors are at risk for this damage. You can reduce your risk by:

- Limiting your time in the sun, especially between 10 a.m. and 2 p.m., when the sun's rays are most intense.

- Wearing clothing to cover skin exposed to the sun—such as long-sleeve shirts, pants, sunglasses, and broad-brim hats. Sun-protective clothing is now available. (The U.S. Food and Drug Administration (FDA) regulates these products only if they are intended to be used for medical purposes.)

- Using broad spectrum sunscreens with a sun-protection factor (SPF) value of 15 or higher regularly and as directed. (Broad spectrum sunscreens offer protection against both UVA and UVB rays, two types of the sun's ultraviolet radiation.)

Always read the label to ensure you use your sunscreen correctly, and ask a healthcare professional before applying sunscreen to infants younger than 6 months.

In general, the FDA recommends that you use broad-spectrum sunscreen with an SPF of 15 or higher, even on cloudy days.

- Apply sunscreen liberally to all uncovered skin, especially your nose, ears, neck, hands, feet, and lips (but avoid putting it inside your mouth and eyes).

- Reapply at least every two hours. Apply more often if you're swimming or sweating. (Read the label for your specific sunscreen. An average-size adult or child needs at least one ounce of sunscreen, about the amount it takes to fill a shot glass, to evenly cover the body.)

- If you don't have much hair, apply sunscreen to the top of your head, or wear a hat.

- No sunscreen completely blocks UV radiation, and other protections are needed, such as protective clothing, sunglasses, and staying in the shade.

- No sunscreen is waterproof.

Note:

- Certain sunscreens have FDA-approved New Drug Applications. Others are marketed under the FDA's over-the-counter (OTC) Drug Review. Sunscreens are available in forms such as lotions, creams, sticks, gels, oils, butters, pastes, and sprays.

- Sunscreen products in forms including wipes, towelettes, powders, body washes, and shampoos that are marketed without an FDA-approved application or outside the FDA's OTC Drug Review remain subject to regulatory action.

How To Read Sunscreen Labels

Although UVB rays are the primary cause of sunburn, both UVA and UVB rays contribute to skin cancer. All sunscreens protect against the sun's UVB rays, but only those that are broad spectrum also protect against UVA rays.

Scientific studies have determined that broad spectrum sunscreens with an SPF of at least 15 can help reduce the risk of sun-induced skin cancer and premature skin aging when used with other sun protective measures, as directed. If you have lighter skin, you may want to use a sunscreen with an SPF higher than 15.

Under the FDA's final regulations:

- Products that pass a broad spectrum test can be labeled "broad spectrum."

- Sunscreens that are not broad spectrum or that lack an SPF of at least 15 must carry a warning: "Skin Cancer/Skin Aging Alert: Spending time in the sun increases your risk of skin cancer and early skin aging. This product has been shown only to help prevent sunburn, not skin cancer or early skin aging."

- Water resistance claims, for 40 or 80 minutes, tell how much time you can expect to get the labeled SPF-level of protection while swimming or sweating.

- Manufacturers may no longer make claims that their sunscreens are "waterproof" or "sweat proof."

- Products may no longer be identified as "sunblocks" or claim instant protection or protection for more than two hours without reapplying.

Risk Factors For Harmful Effects Of UV Radiation

Remember, people of all skin colors are potentially at risk for sunburn and other harmful effects of UV radiation, so always protect yourself. Be especially careful if you have:

- pale skin

- blond, red, or light brown hair

- been treated for skin cancer

- a family member who has had skin cancer

If you take medications, ask your healthcare professional about sun-care precautions. Some medications may increase sun sensitivity. Even on an overcast day, up to 80 percent of the sun's UV rays can get through the clouds. Stay in the shade as much as possible.

Protect Your Eyes With Sunglasses

Sunlight reflecting off sand, water, or even snow, further increases exposure to UV radiation and increases your risk of developing eye problems.

Certain sunglasses can help protect your eyes. When using sunglasses:

- Choose sunglasses labeled with a UVA/UVB rating of 100 percent to get the most UV protection.

- Do not mistake dark-tinted sunglasses as having more UV protection. The darkness of the lens does not indicate its ability to shield your eyes from UV rays. Many sunglasses with light-colored tints, such as green, amber, red, and gray can offer the same UV protection as very dark lenses.

- Children should wear sunglasses that indicate the UV protection level. Toy sunglasses may not have UV protection, so be sure to look for the UV protection label.

- Consider large, wraparound-style frames, which may provide more efficient UV protection because they cover the entire eye-socket.

This is especially important when doing activities around or on water because much of the UV comes from light reflected off the water's surface.

- Understand that pricier sunglasses don't ensure greater UV protection.

- Even if you wear contact lenses, wear sunglasses that offer UV protection.

- Know that sunglasses are the most effective when worn with a wide-brim hat and sunscreen.

Chapter 53

Indoor Tanning And Tanning Products

Intentional UV tanning means exposing your skin to ultraviolet (UV) rays for the purpose of making your skin darker. When the UV rays come from the sun, this behavior is called outdoor tanning. When the UV rays come from a tanning bed, booth, or sunlamp, it is called indoor tanning.

Any change in skin color after UV exposure (whether it is a tan or a burn) is a sign of injury, not health. UV rays from the sun and indoor tanning devices can damage the skin. In response to that damage, the skin makes more melanin, the pigment that gives skin its color, causing it to darken.

Intentional UV tanning does not include the use of cosmetic products such as sunless tanners and bronzers that are designed to make a person look tanned without going out in the sun or using artificial sources of UV rays.

Exposure to ultraviolet (UV) rays while indoor tanning can cause skin cancers including melanoma (the deadliest type of skin cancer), basal cell carcinoma, and squamous cell carcinoma. UV exposure also can cause cataracts and cancers of the eye (ocular melanoma). UV exposure from the sun and from indoor tanning is classified as a human carcinogen (causes cancer in humans) by the International Agency for Research on Cancer (IARC) (part of the World Health Organization(WHO)) and by the U.S. Department of Health and Human Services (HHS).

About This Chapter: Text in this chapter begins with excerpts from "Skin Cancer—Intentional UV Tanning," Centers for Disease Control and Prevention (CDC), April 26, 2017; Text beginning with the heading "Tanning Lamps, Booths, And Beds" is excerpted from "Tanning—Tanning Products," U.S. Food and Drug Administration (FDA), March 29, 2017.

Sunless Tanners And Bronzers

Neither the laws nor the regulations enforced by U.S. Food and Drug Administration (FDA) define the term "sunless tanner." It typically refers to products that provide a tanned appearance without exposure to the sun or other sources of ultraviolet radiation. One commonly used ingredient in these products is dihydroxyacetone (DHA), a color additive that darkens the skin by reacting with amino acids in the skin's surface.

Like the term "sunless tanner," "bronzer" is not defined in either the laws or the regulations enforced by FDA. It is often used to describe a variety of products intended to achieve a temporary tanned appearance. For example, among the products marketed as bronzers are tinted moisturizers and brush-on powders. These produce a temporary effect, similar to other types of makeup, and wash off over time. Some products are marketed with other ingredients in addition to DHA in order to provide a tanned appearance.

(Source: "Sunless Tanners & Bronzers," U.S. Food and Drug Administration (FDA).)

Dangers Of Indoor Tanning

Indoor tanning exposes users to two types of UV rays, UVA and UVB, which damage the skin and can lead to cancer. Indoor tanning is particularly dangerous for younger users; people who begin indoor tanning during adolescence or early adulthood have a higher risk of getting melanoma. This may be due to greater use of indoor tanning among those who begin tanning at earlier ages.

Every time you tan you increase your risk of getting skin cancer, including melanoma. Indoor tanning also:

• Causes premature skin aging, like wrinkles and age spots.

• Changes your skin texture.

• Increases the risk of potentially blinding eye diseases, if eye protection is not used.

The Riskiest Practices

All use of tanning beds increases the risk of skin cancer. Certain practices are especially dangerous. These include:

• Failing to wear the goggles provided, which can lead to short- and long-term eye injury.

- Starting with long exposures (close to the maximum time for the particular tanning bed), which can lead to burning. Because sunburn takes 6 to 48 hours to develop, you may not realize your skin is burned until it's too late.
- Failing to follow manufacturer-recommended exposure times on the label for your skin type.
- Tanning while using certain medications or cosmetics that may make you more sensitive to UV rays. Talk to your doctor or pharmacist first.

(Source: "Indoor Tanning: The Risks Of Ultraviolet Rays," U.S. Food and Drug Administration (FDA).)

Facts About Indoor Tanning

Tanning indoors is not safer than tanning in the sun. Indoor tanning and tanning outside are both dangerous. Although indoor tanning devices operate on a timer, the exposure to UV rays can vary based on the age and type of light bulbs. Indoor tanning is designed to give you high levels of UV radiation in a short time. You can get a burn from tanning indoors, and even a tan indicates damage to your skin.

A base tan is not a safe tan. A tan is the body's response to injury from UV rays. A base tan does little to protect you from future damage to your skin caused by UV exposure. In fact, people who indoor tan are more likely to report getting sunburned.

Indoor tanning is not a safe way to get vitamin D. Although it is important to get enough vitamin D, the safest way to do so is through what you eat. Tanning harms your skin, and the amount of UV exposure you need to get enough vitamin D is hard to measure because it is different for every person and also varies with the weather, latitude, altitude, and more.

National Statistics On Indoor Tanning

According to the 2015 Youth Risk Behavior Surveillance System (YRBSS), some teens are indoor tanning, including:

- 7 percent of all high school students.
- 11 percent of high school girls.
- 16 percent of girls in the 12th grade.
- 15 percent of white high school girls.

Tanning Lamps, Booths, And Beds

Tanning lamps have become a popular method of maintaining a year-round tan, but their effects can be as dangerous as tanning outdoors.

Like the sun, the lamps used in tanning booths and beds emit ultraviolet (UV) radiation. While most lamps emit both UVA and UVB radiation, some emit only UVA.

Some advocates argue that artificial tanning is less dangerous because the intensity of light and the time spent tanning are controlled. There is limited evidence to support these claims. On the other hand, sunlamps may be more dangerous than the sun because they can be used at a constant intensity every day of the year—something that is unlikely for the sun because of winter weather and cloud cover. Sunlamps can also be more dangerous because people tend to expose more of their bodies to sunlamps than when outdoors.

Given the risk from tanning, the U.S. Food and Drug Administration (FDA) in 2014 reclassified the devices as class II, requiring special controls and premarket review. The special controls require, among others, that labeling be included on sunlamp products stating that the products should not be used by anyone younger than 18, and will require specific warnings be included in certain promotional materials for sunlamp products and UV lamps.

Because people under age 18 are especially at risk of skin cancer from use of these devices, the FDA is now proposing to restrict tanning facility operators from allowing use of the device by consumers under 18 years old, and operators must obtain a signed, FDA-prescribed risk acknowledgement certification before use that states that they have been informed of the risks to health that may result from use of sunlamp products.

Using tanning lamps, booths, or beds:

If you use indoor tanning equipment, follow these steps to reduce the dangers of UV exposure.

- Don't use indoor tanning equipment if you are under 18 years old.

- Be sure to wear the goggles provided, making sure they fit snugly and are not cracked.

- Start slowly and use short exposure times to buildup a tan over time.

- Don't use the maximum exposure time the first time you tan because you could get burned, and burns are thought to be related to melanoma.

- Follow manufacturer-recommended exposure times for your skin type. Check the label for exposure times.

- Stick to your time limit.

- After a tan is developed, tan no more than once a week. Depending on your skin type, you may even be able to maintain your tan with one exposure every 2–3 weeks.

- Even if you follow these safety instructions, you are still at risk for skin cancer if you use indoor UV tanning devices.

Because sunburn takes 6 to 48 hours to develop, you may not realize your skin is burned until it is too late.

FDA is proposing to revise its electronic product performance standard (21 CFR 1040.20) for sunlamp products. All sunlamp products must have a warning label, an accurate timer, an emergency stop control, and include an exposure schedule and protective goggles. The proposed revision updates and strengthens these requirements. The revised warning label would strengthen the language and make it easier to read.

You should not use a tanning bed or lamp if:

- You are under 18 years old.

- You sunburn easily and do not tan. Skin that does not tan in the sun will probably not tan under a sunlamp and is at higher risk of developing skin cancer.

- You or your family has a history of skin cancer.

- You get frequent cold sores. UV radiation may cause them to appear more frequently due to immune system suppression.

- You are taking medicines that can make you more sensitive to UV rays. Check with your doctor or pharmacist.

- You have skin lesions or open wounds.

Sunless Tanning Sprays And Lotions

Sunless tanning delivers a faux glow by coating your skin with the chemical dihydroxyacetone (DHA). DHA interacts with the dead surface cells in the epidermis to darken skin color and simulate a tan, and the result usually lasts for several days.

While the FDA allows DHA to be "externally applied" for skin coloring, there are restrictions on its use. DHA should not be inhaled, ingested, or exposed to areas covered by mucous membranes including the lips, nose, and areas in and around the eye (from the top of the cheek to above the eyebrow) because the risks, if any, are unknown.

Most sunless tanning sprays and lotions do not contain a skin protecting sunscreen. Make sure you apply an even coat of sunscreen to all exposed skin at least 30 minutes before going outdoors.

The FDA is aware that some tanning salons sell packages with both sunless tanning spray and UV tanning. The risk of combining exposure to UV radiation from either the sun or indoor tanning devices followed by sunless tanning sprays (or vice versa) is unknown in humans.

Using Sunless Tanners

Before using a sunless tanning booth, ask the tanning salon these questions to make sure you will be protected:

- Will my eyes and the area surrounding them be protected?

- Will my nose, mouth, and ears be protected?

- Will I be protected from inhaling the tanning spray through my nose or mouth?

If the answer to any of these questions is "no," look for another salon. Otherwise, you are putting yourself at risk for exposure to chemicals with potentially dangerous effects.

You should also take precautions if you're applying a self-tanner at home. Most self-tanners contain the same DHA used in sunless tanning salons. Self-tanners are available in many forms, including lotions, creams, and sprays that you apply and let soak into your skin. Follow the directions on the self-tanner label carefully and take care not to get the self-tanner in your eyes, nose, or mouth.

Tanning Pills

You may have seen ads that promise to give you a too-good-to-be-true golden glow just by swallowing a pill. These so-called tanning pills are unsafe and none are approved by the FDA.

Some tanning pills contain the color additive canthaxanthin. When large amounts of canthaxanthin are ingested, it can turn the skin a range of colors from orange to brown. It can also cause serious health problems including liver damage; hives; and an eye disorder called canthaxanthin retinopathy, in which yellow deposits form in the retinas.

Chapter 54

Risks Of Tanning

Sunburn

Sunburn, also called erythema, is one of the most obvious signs of ultraviolet (UV) exposure and skin damage. Often marked by redness and peeling (usually after a few days), sunburn is a form of short-term skin damage.

Why It Happens

When UV rays reach your skin, they damage cells in the epidermis. In response, your immune system increases blood flow to the affected areas. The increased blood flow is what gives sunburn its characteristic redness and makes the skin feel warm to the touch. At the same time, the damaged skin cells release chemicals that send messages through the body until they are translated as a painful burning sensation by the brain.

White blood cells, which help protect you from infection and disease, attack and remove the damaged skin cells. It is this process of removing damaged cells that can cause sunburned skin to itch and peel.

Symptoms

The earliest signs of sunburn are skin that looks flushed, is tender or painful, or gives off more heat than normal. Unfortunately, if your skin tone is medium to dark you may not notice any obvious physical signs until several hours later. It can take 6–48 hours for the full effects of sunburn to appear.

About This Chapter: This chapter includes text excerpted from "The Risks Of Tanning," U.S. Food and Drug Administration (FDA), October 14, 2015.

Treatment

The American Academy of Dermatology (AAD) recommends treating mild sunburn with cool baths, over-the-counter hydrocortisone creams, and aspirin to ease pain and swelling.

Severe sunburn should be treated as a medical emergency and examined by a doctor right away. Severe sunburn is often characterized by a large area of red, blistered skin with a headache, fever, or chills.

The Bottom Line

Sunburn can be a very painful effect of UV exposure. Studies have shown a link between severe sunburn and melanoma, the deadliest form of skin cancer. Pay careful attention to protecting yourself from UV rays.

Sun Tan

There is no such thing as a safe tan. The increase in skin pigment, called melanin, which causes the tan color change in your skin is a sign of damage.

Why It Happens

Once skin is exposed to UV radiation, it increases the production of melanin in an attempt to protect the skin from further damage. Melanin is the same pigment that colors your hair, eyes, and skin. The increase in melanin may cause your skin tone to darken over the next 48 hours.

Symptoms

Skin tones that are capable of developing a tan, typically skin types II through V, will probably darken in tone within two days.

The Bottom Line

Evidence suggests that tanning greatly increases your risk of developing skin cancer. And, contrary to popular belief, getting a tan will not protect your skin from sunburn or other skin damage. The extra melanin in tanned skin provides a sun-protection factor (SPF) of about 2 to 4; far below the minimum recommended SPF of 15.

Premature Aging

Sometimes referred to as "photoaging," premature aging is the result of unprotected UV exposure. It takes the form of leathery, wrinkled skin, and dark spots.

Why It Happens

Although the causes of premature aging are not always clear, unprotected exposure to harmful UV rays break down the collagen and elastin fibers in healthy young skin, and cause wrinkles and loosened folds. Frequent sunburns or hours spent tanning can result in a permanent darkening of the skin, dark spots, and a leathery texture.

Symptoms

- Wrinkles
- Dark spots
- Leathery skin

Treatment

A dermatologist or plastic surgeon can develop a treatment plan based on your needs. Treatments can include chemical peels, dermabrasion, and skin fillers.

The Bottom Line

Premature aging is a long-term side effect of UV exposure, meaning it may not show on your skin until many years after you have had a sunburn or suntan. Avoiding UV exposure is essential to maintaining healthy skin.

Skin Cancer

There are two main types of skin cancer:

- Melanoma
- Nonmelanoma

Melanoma is the less common, but more dangerous form of skin cancer, and accounts for most of the deaths due to skin cancer each year. Melanoma is cancer that begins in the epidermal cells that produce melanin (melanocytes). According to the American Cancer Society (ACS) melanoma is almost always curable when detected in its early stages.

Nonmelanomas (basal cell and squamous cell carcinomas) occur in the basal or squamous cells located at the base of the epidermis, both inside and outside the body. Nonmelanomas often develop in sun-exposed areas of the body, including the face, ears, neck, lips, and the backs of the hands.

Why It Happens

Predisposition to skin cancer can be hereditary, meaning it is passed through the generations of a family through genes. There is also strong evidence suggesting that exposure to UV rays, both UVA and UVB, can cause skin cancer.

UV radiation may promote skin cancer in two different ways:

- By damaging the DNA in skin cells, causing the skin to grow abnormally and develop benign or malignant growths.

- By weakening the immune system and compromising the body's natural defenses against aggressive cancer cells.

Symptoms

Performing regular self skin cancer exams is a good way to protect yourself against skin cancer. The following are possible signs of skin cancer, and should be checked by a doctor.

- Any changes on the skin, especially in the size or color of a mole, birthmark, or other dark pigmentation

- Unexplained scaliness, oozing, or bleeding on the skin's surface

- A spot on the skin that suddenly feels itchy, tender, or painful

Treatment

Skin cancer treatment varies depending on the type and severity of the cancer. Your doctor will develop a treatment plan based on your needs.

The Bottom Line

According to the American Cancer Society (ACS), most of the more than one million skin cancers diagnosed each year in the United States are considered sun-related. Skin cancer occurs in people of all skin tones, though it is less common in those with darker skin tones. Assessing your risk with the help of your doctor, protecting your skin, and performing regular skin cancer checks are the best methods of prevention.

Actinic Or Solar Keratoses

A fourth type of growth, actinic or solar keratoses, is a concern because it can progress into cancer. Actinic keratoses are considered the earliest stage in the development of skin cancer, and are caused by long-term exposure to sunlight. They are the most common premalignant skin condition, occurring in more than 5 million Americans each year.

Symptoms

Actinic or solar keratoses share some of the symptoms of skin cancer. Look for raised, rough-textured, or scaly bumps that occur in areas that have been sunburned or tanned.

Treatment

Most cases of actinic keratoses are easily treated in a dermatologist's office by removing them with liquid nitrogen or chemical peels.

The Bottom Line

Actinic or solar keratoses are the most common premalignant skin condition. Check with your doctor if you find any suspicious-looking bumps.

Eye Damage: Photokeratitis

Photokeratitis can be thought of as a sunburn of the cornea. It is caused by intense UVC/UVB exposure of the eye. Photokeratitis is also called "snow blindness" because many people develop this condition at high altitudes in a snowy environment where the reflections of UVB are high. This condition can also be produced by exposure to intense artificial sources of UVC/UVB, like broken mercury vapor lamps, or certain types of tanning lamps.

Symptoms

- Tearing
- Pain
- Swollen eyelids
- A feeling of sand in the eye
- Hazy or decreased vision

Treatment

Consult your doctor if you have any of these symptoms. Your doctor can prescribe a topical solution which will aid your cornea in healing. Since the cornea usually heals in 24 to 48 hours, the symptoms are not long-lasting.

Eye Damage: Cataracts

Cataracts are one form of eye damage that research has shown may increase with UV exposure. Clouding of the natural lens of the eye causing decreased vision and possible blindness are all effects of cataracts.

Other types of eye damage include cancer around the eyes, macular degeneration, and irregular tissue growth that can block vision (pterygium).

Symptoms

Consult your doctor if you experience any of the following symptoms.

- Clouded or spotty vision

- Pain or soreness in and around the eyes

Treatment

Cataracts can be surgically removed.

The Bottom Line

Wearing sun protection gear such as a wide-brimmed hat and sunglasses with 100 percent UV protection can help decrease the risks of eye damage.

Immune System Suppression

According to the World Health Organization (WHO), all people, regardless of skin color, are vulnerable to the effects of immune suppression. Overexposure to UV radiation may suppress proper functioning of the body's immune system and the skin's natural defenses, increasing sensitivity to sunlight, diminishing the effects of immunizations or causing reactions to certain medications.

In people who have been treated for an infection of the Herpes simplex virus, sun exposure can weaken the immune system so that it can no longer keep the virus under control. This results in reactivation of the infection and recurring cold sores.

Chapter 55

Tattoos And Tattoo Removal

Tattoos are more popular than ever. According to a Harris Poll, about 3 in 10 (or 29%) people surveyed have at least one tattoo. The U.S. Food and Drug Administration (FDA) is also seeing reports of people developing infections from contaminated tattoo inks, as well as adverse reactions to the inks themselves.

Over the years, the FDA has received hundreds of adverse event reports involving tattoos: 363 from 2004–2016.

Should I Be Concerned About Unsafe Practices, Or The Tattoo Ink Itself?

Both. While you can get serious infections from unhygienic practices and equipment that isn't sterile, infections can also result from ink that was contaminated with bacteria or mold. Using nonsterile water to dilute the pigments (ingredients that add color) is a common culprit, although not the only one.

There's no sure-fire way to tell if the ink is safe. An ink can be contaminated even if the container is sealed or the label says the product is sterile.

What Is In Tattoo Ink?

Published research has reported that some inks contain pigments used in printer toner or in car paint. FDA has not approved any pigments for injection into the skin for cosmetic purposes.

About This Chapter: Text in this chapter begins with excerpts from "Think Before You Ink: Are Tattoos Safe?" U.S. Food And Drug Administration (FDA), May 10, 2017; Text beginning with the heading "Lasers, Dermabrasion, And Other Methods For Tattoo Removal" is excerpted from "Tattoo Removal: Options And Results," U.S. Food And Drug Administration (FDA), June 28, 2017.

FDA reviews reports of adverse reactions or infections from consumers and healthcare providers. We may learn about outbreaks from the state authorities who oversee tattoo parlors.

How About Henna?

You may have seen temporary tattoos that an artist paints on using a dye like henna. These can cause an allergic reaction even a couple of weeks later. Black henna can cause dangerous reactions in some people. And no henna should ever be injected under your skin.

(Source: "Tattoos And Piercing," girlshealth.gov, Office on Women's Health (OWH).)

What Kinds Of Reactions May Happen After Getting A Tattoo?

You might notice a rash—redness or bumps—in the area of your tattoo, and you could develop a fever.

More aggressive infections may cause high fever, shaking, chills, and sweats. Treating such infections might require a variety of antibiotics—possibly for months—or even hospitalization and/or surgery. A rash may also mean you're having an allergic reaction. And because the inks are permanent, the reaction may persist.

Contact your healthcare professional if you have any concerns.

Can Scar Tissue Buildup After Getting A Tattoo?

Scar tissue may form when you get a tattoo, or you could develop "granulomas," small knots or bumps that may form around material that the body perceives as foreign. If you tend to get keloids—scars that grow beyond normal boundaries—you may develop the same kind of reaction to the tattoo.

What Do I Need To Know About Magnetic Resonance Imaging (MRI) If I Get A Tattoo?

Some people may have swelling or burning in the tattoo when they have magnetic resonance imaging (MRI), although this happens rarely and does not last long. Let your healthcare professional know that you have a tattoo before an MRI is ordered.

What About Do-It-Yourself Tattoo Inks And Kits?

Inks and kits sold as "do-it-yourself" to consumers have been associated with infections and allergic reactions. FDA is also concerned that consumers may not know how to control and avoid all sources of contamination.

Could Other Problems Occur Later On?

Although research is ongoing at FDA and elsewhere, there are still a lot of questions about the long-term effects of the pigments, other ingredients, and possible contaminants in tattoo inks. FDA has received reports of bad reactions to tattoo inks right after tattooing and even years later. You also might become allergic to other products, such as hair dyes, if your tattoo contains p-phenylenediamene (PPD).

Then there's tattoo removal. We don't know the short- or long-term consequences of how pigments break down after laser treatment. However, we do know some tattoo removal procedures may leave permanent scarring.

If I Get A Tattoo And Develop An Infection Or Other Reaction, What Would I Do?

First, contact your healthcare professional.

Second, notify the tattoo artist so he or she can identify the ink and avoid using it again. Ask for the brand, color, and any lot or batch number of the ink or diluent to help determine the source of the problem and how to treat it.

Third, whether you're a consumer, tattoo artist, or healthcare professional, tell FDA. Provide as much detail as possible about the ink and your reaction and outcome. Reports from consumers are one of our most important sources of safety information.

Removing Tattoos May Be Harder Than You Think

So think before you ink. Consider the risks.

Remember, too, that removing a tattoo is a painstaking process, and complete removal without scarring may be impossible.

If you do decide to get a tattoo, make sure the tattoo parlor and artist comply with state and local laws.

Lasers, Dermabrasion, And Other Methods For Tattoo Removal

Tattoos are meant to be permanent. Artists create tattoos by using an electrically powered machine that moves a needle up and down to inject ink into the skin, penetrating the epidermis, or outer layer, and depositing a drop of ink into the dermis, the second layer of skin. The cells of the dermis are more stable compared with those of the epidermis, so the ink will mostly stay in place for a person's lifetime.

An effective and safe way to remove tattoos is through laser surgery, performed by a dermatologist who specializes in tattoo removal, says FDA's Mehmet Kosoglu, Ph.D. With laser removal, pulses of high-intensity laser energy pass through the epidermis and are selectively absorbed by the tattoo pigment. The laser breaks the pigment into smaller particles, which may be metabolized or excreted by the body, or transported to and stored in lymph nodes or other tissues, Kosoglu explains.

The type of laser used to remove a tattoo depends on the tattoo's pigment colors, he adds. Because every color of ink absorbs different wavelengths of light, multi-colored tattoos may require the use of multiple lasers. Lighter colors such as green, red, and yellow are the hardest colors to remove, while blue and black are the easiest.

Generally speaking, just one laser treatment won't do the trick. According to the American Academy of Dermatology (AAD), the procedure requires multiple treatments (typically six to 10) depending on a tattoo's size and colors, and requires a few weeks of healing time between procedures.

Kosoglu says that pulsed lasers have been used to remove tattoos for more than 20 years. However, it can be a painstaking process. "Complete removal, with no scarring, is sometimes not possible," Kosoglu notes.

Other methods include dermabrasion—actually "sanding" away the top layer of skin—and excision, cutting away the area of the tattoo and then sewing the skin back together.

Pain And Side Effects Of Laser Tattoo Removal

Does tattoo removal hurt? "That depends on a person's pain threshold," Kosoglu says. Some people compare the sensation of laser removal to being spattered with drops of hot bacon grease or snapping a thin rubber band against the skin. A trained dermatologist will be able to adjust the treatment to the patient's comfort level.

Some side effects may include pinpoint bleeding, redness, or soreness, none of which should last for long. Another possible side effect of tattoo removal is scarring.

Luke says that these laser devices are cleared for use by, or under the supervision of, a healthcare professional. The removal procedure requires using the correct type of laser, understanding the reaction of tissue to laser, and knowing how to treat the area after the procedure.

"If you have any concerns about having a tattoo removed, it's a good idea to consult your dermatologist, who is knowledgeable about laser treatments," Luke concludes.

Bye-Bye, Tattoo?

Sometimes it's just not possible to remove a tattoo. Other times it can be cut off or sanded down. Laser removal is an option, but it can take months and lots of money. And beware of tattoo removal creams that you can buy online. There is no proof they work, and they can cause dangerous skin reactions.

(Source: "Tattoos And Piercing," girlshealth.gov, Office on Women's Health (OWH).)

Chapter 56

Piercings

Piercings are body decorations that go back to ancient times. Body piercing involves making a hole in the skin so that you can insert jewelry. This is often in the earlobe, but can be in other parts of the body.

The health risks of piercings include:

- Allergic reactions

- Keloids, a type of scar that forms during healing

- Infections, such as hepatitis

To reduce the risks, make sure that the facility is clean, safe, and has a good reputation. Proper sterilization of the equipment is important. Be sure to follow the instructions on caring for your skin.

Holes from piercing usually close up if you no longer wear the jewelry.

Tips To Avoid Piercing Problems

Some people think piercings and tattoos look cool. In fact, some people call them body art. But body art can be risky to get and hard to get rid of. Make your decision carefully, and follow the advice below to protect your precious body.

About This Chapter: Text in this chapter begins with excerpts from "Piercing And Tattoos," MedlinePlus, National Institutes of Health (NIH), January 26, 2017; Text beginning with the heading "Tips To Avoid Piercing Problems" is excerpted from "Tattoos And Piercing," girlshealth.gov, Office On Women's Health (OWH), April 15, 2014.

Because piercing involves making a hole in your body with a needle, there's a chance that germs may enter your body through that hole. In addition, you can have an allergic reaction to jewelry that's used in piercing.

Consider these tips to avoid piercing problems:

- **Never let a friend pierce your ear or anything else.** You want clean conditions and someone who has been trained.

- **Make sure your piercing is done with a new, clean needle.** Sharing dirty needles puts you at risk for serious infections, like hepatitis B.

- **Make sure the person doing the piercing wears gloves.**

- **If the person piercing your ears is going to use a piercing gun, a single-use piercing gun is safest.** Reusable piercing guns that use sterilized disposable cassettes may be ok, but some experts say any reusable guns should be avoided.

- **To avoid an allergic reaction, look for jewelry made of titanium, 14-karat gold, or surgical-grade steel.**

- **Ask how long it will take to heal.** Some parts of your body can take months to heal.

- **Think carefully about mouth piercings.** Infections are common, and tongue jewelry can damage your front teeth and gums. You may want to get a doctor's advice before piercing your mouth (or any part of your body that is sensitive or that doesn't heal easily).

- **Make sure you know how to take care of the piercing.** If it gets infected, see a doctor right away (but it's probably ok to wait until the next day if you see the infection at night).

- **Beware of stretching a piercing.** Sometimes people make a small piercing into a large hole, usually in the earlobe. Possible problems from stretching include infections and scarring, the lobe splitting open, and needing surgery if you want to close the hole.

Chapter 57

Hair Loss: Alopecia Areata

What Is Alopecia Areata?

Alopecia areata is a disease that affects the hair follicles, which are part of the skin from which hairs grow. In most cases, hair falls out in small, round patches about the size of a quarter. Many people with the disease get only a few bare patches. Some people may lose more hair. Rarely, the disease causes total loss of hair on the head or complete loss of hair on the head, face, and body.

Who Gets Alopecia Areata?

Anyone can have alopecia areata. It often begins in childhood. There is a slightly increased risk of having the disease if you have a close family member with the disease.

What Causes Alopecia Areata?

Alopecia areata is an autoimmune disease. Normally the immune system protects the body against infection and disease. In an autoimmune disease, the body's immune system mistakenly attacks some part of your own body. In alopecia areata, the immune system attacks the hair follicles.

The cause is not known. Scientists think that a person's genes may play a role. For people whose genes put them at risk for the disease, some type of trigger starts the attack on the hair follicles. The triggers may be a virus or something in the person's environment.

About This Chapter: This chapter includes text excerpted from "Fast Facts About Alopecia Areata," National Institute Of Arthritis And Musculoskeletal And Skin Diseases (NIAMS), April 2015.

Will My Hair Ever Grow Back?

There is every chance that your hair will grow back, but it may fall out again. No one can tell you when it might fall out or grow back. You may lose more hair, or your hair loss may stop. The hair you have lost may or may not grow back. Even a person who has lost all of his hair may grow all of his hair back. The disease varies from person to person.

How Is Alopecia Areata Treated?

There is no cure for alopecia areata. There are no drugs approved to treat it. Doctors may use medicines approved for other diseases to help hair grow back.

However, none of these treatments prevent new patches of hair loss or cure the disease. Talk to your doctor about the treatment that is best for you.

How Will Alopecia Areata Affect My Life?

Alopecia areata does not make you feel pain and does not make you feel sick. You can't give it to others. People who have the disease are, for the most part, healthy in other ways. Alopecia areata will not shorten your life, and it should not affect activities such as going to school, working, marrying, raising a family, playing sports, and exercising.

How Can I Cope With The Effects Of This Disease

Living with hair loss can be hard. There are many things you can do to cope with the effects of this disease, including:

- Learning as much as you can about the disease.
- Talking with others who are dealing with the disease.
- Learning to value yourself for who you are, not for how much hair you have or don't have.
- Talking with a counselor, if necessary, to help build a positive self-image.

Here are some things you can use to reduce the physical dangers or discomforts of lost hair:

- Use sunscreens for the scalp, face, and all exposed skin.
- Wear eyeglasses (or sunglasses) to protect eyes from sun, and from dust and debris, when eyebrows or eyelashes are missing.

- Wear wigs, caps, or scarves to protect the scalp from the sun and keep the head warm.

- Apply antibiotic ointment inside the nostrils to help keep germs out of the nose when nostril hair is missing.

Here are some things you can do to reduce the disease's effects on your looks:

- Try wearing a wig, hairpiece, scarf, or cap.

- Use a hair-colored powder, cream, or crayon applied to the scalp for small patches of hair loss to make the hair loss less obvious.

- Use an eyebrow pencil to mask missing eyebrows.

Chapter 58

Unwanted Hair: Removing Hair Safely

Laser Hair Removal

In this method, a laser destroys hair follicles with heat. Sometimes it is recommended that a topical anesthetic product be used before a laser hair removal procedure, to minimize pain. In these cases, U.S. Food and Drug Administration (FDA) recommends that consumers discuss with a medical professional the circumstances under which the cream should be used and whether the use is appropriate.

Those who decide to use a skin-numbing product should follow the directions of a healthcare provider and consider using a product that contains the lowest amount of anesthetic drugs possible. FDA's Center for Drug Evaluation and Research (CDER) has received reports of serious and life-threatening side effects after use of large amounts of skin-numbing products for laser hair removal.

Side effects of laser hair removal can include blistering, discoloration after treatment, swelling, redness, and scarring. Sunlight should be avoided during healing after the procedure.

Epilators: Needle, Electrolysis, And Tweezers

Needle epilators introduce a fine wire close to the hair shaft, under the skin, and into the hair follicle. An electric current travels down the wire and destroys the hair root at the bottom of the follicle, and the loosened hair is removed with tweezers.

About This Chapter: This chapter includes text excerpted from "Removing Hair Safely," U.S. Food And Drug Administration (FDA), August 28, 2015.

Medical electrolysis devices destroy hair growth with a shortwave radio frequency after a thin probe is placed in the hair follicle. Risks from these methods include infection from an unsterile needle and scarring from improper technique. Electrolysis is considered a permanent hair removal method since it destroys the hair follicle. It requires a series of appointments over a period of time.

Tweezer epilators also use electric current to remove hair. The tweezers grasp the hair close to the skin, and energy is applied at the tip of the tweezer. There is no body of significant information establishing the effectiveness of the tweezer epilator to permanently remove hair.

Depilatories

Available in gel, cream, lotion, aerosol, and roll-on forms, depilatories are highly alkaline (or, in some cases, acidic) formulations that affect the protein structure of the hair, causing it to dissolve into a jelly like mass that the user can easily wipe from the skin. Consumers should carefully follow instructions and heed all warnings on the product label.

For example, manufacturers typically recommend conducting a preliminary skin test for allergic reaction and irritation. Depilatories should not be used for eyebrows or around eyes or on inflamed or broken skin.

FDA's Office of Cosmetics and Colors has received reports of burns, blisters, stinging, itchy rashes, and skin peeling associated with depilatories and other types of cosmetic hair removers.

Waxing, Sugaring, And Threading

Unlike chemical depilatories that remove hair at the skin's surface, these methods pluck hairs out of the follicle, below the surface.

With waxing, a layer of melted wax is applied to the skin and allowed to harden. (Cold waxes, which are soft at room temperature, allow the user to skip the steps of melting and hardening.) It is then pulled off quickly in the opposite direction of the hair growth, taking the uprooted hair with it. Labeling of waxes may caution that these products should not be used by people with diabetes and circulatory problems. Waxes should not be used over varicose veins, moles, or warts. Waxes also shouldn't be used on eyelashes, the nose, ears, or on nipples, genital areas, or on irritated, chapped, or sunburned skin. As with chemical depilatories, it can be a good idea to do a preliminary test on a small area for allergic reaction or irritation.

Sugaring is similar to waxing. A heated sugar mixture is spread on the skin, sometimes covered with a strip of fabric, and then lifted off to remove hair. Threading is an ancient technique in which a loop of thread is rotated across the skin to pluck the hair. All of these techniques may cause skin irritation and infection.

Shaving

Shaving hair only when it's wet, and shaving in the direction in which the hairs lie can help lessen skin irritation and cuts. It's important to use a clean razor with a sharp blade. Contrary to popular belief, shaving does not change the texture, color, or growth rate of hair. Razors and electric shavers are under the jurisdiction of the Consumer Product Safety Commission (CPSC).

Chapter 59

Foot Care For A Lifetime

Caring For Your Insensitive Feet

The loss of protective sensation puts you at a high risk for injury, permanent deformity, and even amputation. Following the guidelines of this chapter will help you protect your feet and greatly reduce the chances of foot problems that commonly occur with neuropathy. Regular foot exams by your footcare specialist, daily self-inspection, and wearing protective footwear are the keys to keeping your feet healthy. It is important that you become familiar with the information in this chapter and begin to put it into practice so that these principles will become habits in your daily routine. After reading this chapter, please discuss any questions or concerns you have with your footcare specialist. This will eliminate any confusion and you can plan together for your routine footcare.

Daily Foot Care

Cleaning Your Feet

- Check the water temperature with your hand or elbow to make sure the bath water is a safe temperature. A safe temperature is below 110°F (42–43°C).

- Wash your feet with warm (NOT HOT), soapy water.

- Avoid soaking your feet. Soaking your feet for prolonged periods of time can actually dry the skin.

About This Chapter: This chapter includes text excerpted from "Foot Care For A Lifetime," Health Resources and Services Administration (HRSA), January 2013. Reviewed August 2017.

- While you are washing, do a thorough inspection of your feet. Rinse with warm (NOT HOT), clean water.

- Dry your feet carefully, especially between your toes.

- Apply fragrance free and alcohol free moisturizing lotion immediately after cleaning your feet, but DO NOT put lotion between your toes. Keeping the area between the toes too moist may cause skin breakdown.

Toenail Care

Toenails need care on a regular basis because long or thick nails can press on neighboring toes and cause open sores. It is best to consult a footcare specialist before attempting to cut your own toenails. If you or a family member cuts your toenails, please follow the tips below.

Nail Trimming Tips

- Trim toenails straight across.

- DO NOT cut into the corners of the nail/toe. This can cause an ingrown toenail.

- Use a nail file or Emory board to gently round the edges of the nail.

- NEVER use knives, scissors or razor blades to trim your toenails.

Daily Self-Inspection

The single most important thing you can do to protect your feet is daily self-inspection. Finding problems early and getting help when the problem is small can prevent permanent damage and deformity to your feet. Contact your footcare specialist immediately if you see a problem on your foot, no matter how small it may seem.

When To Inspect

- Before you put on your socks and shoes

- After you take off your socks and shoes

- After you take a bath or shower

- At regular intervals throughout the day

Inspection Tips

- Check between all of your toes. These areas are not generally visible and are often overlooked.

- If you cannot see the bottom of your foot, use a mirror or ask for help from family members or friends.

What To Look For

- Blisters, cuts or scratches can lead to infection if ignored.

- Color changes (blue, bright red or white spots): Color changes can be a sign that the skin is damaged.

- Areas of excessive dryness can crack and allow bacteria to enter the skin.

- Callus or corns are signs of excessive pressure and need to be addressed immediately.

- Swelling can be a sign of injury to the soft tissue or bone and should be brought to the attention of your footcare specialist immediately.

Self-Test Foot Screening

Every person who has neuropathy should have a foot screen. An individual who can feel the filament in the selected sites should not develop foot ulcers associated with neuropathy. Follow the instructions below to determine the level of sensation in your feet.

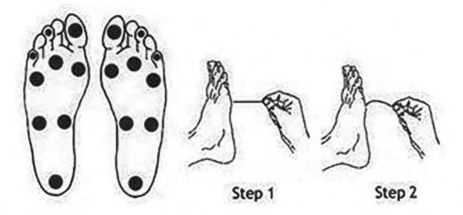

Step 1   Step 2

Figure 59.1. Self-Test Foot Screening

1. Hold the filament by the paper handle as shown in step 1.

2. Use a smooth motion to touch the filament to the skin on your foot. Touch the filament along the side of and NOT directly on an ulcer, callus, or scar. Touch the filament to your skin for 1–2 seconds. Push hard enough to make the filament bend as shown in step 2.

3. Touch the filament to both of your feet in the sites circled in red on the drawing above. Place a (+) in the circle if you can feel the filament at that site and a (-) if you cannot feel the filament at that site.

4. The filament is reusable. After use, wipe with an alcohol swab.

5. If you are unable to feel even one of the areas marked in red, see your footcare specialist as soon as possible. You may have a loss of protective sensation.

Shoes And Socks

When your feet have a loss of protective sensation, the shoes (and socks) you wear can either help you to live a healthy and productive life, or can contribute to repeated open sores that may gradually lead to amputation. No single type or style of shoe is appropriate for everyone. People with insensitive feet have special footwear needs that must be addressed by a footcare specialist in order to prevent ulcers caused by shoes that don't fit properly. The following information is provided to help you make wise choices in the shoes you select and wear every day.

Selecting Shoes

- Without protective sensation, it is difficult for you to know if the shoe is fitting correctly. You may be tempted to choose a shoe that is too tight because it may "feel" better. DO NOT rely on your judgment or feeling as you select your shoes.

- DO NOT choose a shoe just because it is intended for use in patients with neuropathy.

- Select a shoe based on the recommendation of your footcare specialist. Select a shoe that reflects the measured size, shape, and special needs of your feet.

- Select a shoe made of real leather or stretchable material so it will accommodate your foot; or is able to be modified to accommodate your foot.

- Let your footcare specialist check the fit of the shoe BEFORE you wear it so you can return it if you need a different size or style. Check the return policy before purchasing new shoes.

Fitting Shoes

- DO NOT purchase a shoe based on the size you've always worn. There is no size standard for shoes (i.e., size 8D with one manufacturer is different than another manufacturer).

- A properly fitting shoe should have the following characteristics:

- At least 1 inch (a thumb width) between the longest toe and the end of the shoe for proper length.

- Be able to pinch some material at the sides or top of the shoe for proper width.

- The shape of the shoe should match the shape of the foot.

- This can be measured by removing the insert of the shoe and tracing it onto a piece of paper. Then place your foot on the drawing of the insert and trace your foot. Compare the two tracings and see if the shape of the insert matches that of your foot, and if your foot fits within the boundaries of the insert.

Wearing Shoes

- Always check the inside of your shoe before putting them on and after taking them off your feet. Make this a habit every time you put on and take off your shoes.

- Break-in new shoes gradually over several days. Never assume the shoes are safe to wear for an extended time when they are new. Begin with one hour in the morning and one hour in the afternoon, checking your feet after each use. If there are no problems, increase it daily until you can wear them throughout the day without harming your feet.

- Shoes will generally need replacing at least once every year. If you have Medicare Part B and require special footwear, talk to your doctor to see if you qualify for insurance assistance with the purchase of your special footwear.

- Keep your shoes clean and good repair.

- Make sure your footcare specialist checks your shoes every time you have a check-up.

Socks

Socks can either protect or harm the insensitive foot. If socks are loose and wrinkled within the shoe, there is potential for localized pressure that can harm your foot.

A good pair of socks:

- Should provide a good fit and have enough elastic to stay up on the leg.

- Should not have heavy seams that can cause added pressure on the toes.

- Should be white in color so blood or drainage is visible from a blister or ulcer should one occur.

- Always wear socks with your shoes. Socks provide a protective barrier between your skin and your shoe and may prevent skin breakdown.

Footcare Warnings!

- DO NOT use heating pads, electric blankets or hot water bottles. When your feet are sensitive, you can burn them easily without knowing it.

- DO NOT use harsh chemicals on your skin such as callus or corn removers, Hydrogen Peroxide, Alcohol, and Betadine.

- DO NOT use knives, scissors, or razor blades to trim your toenails or callus.

- NEVER go barefoot... not even in the bath or shower. Wear a shower sandal or shower shoe to protect your feet from the hard surface of the tub/shower. Ask your footcare specialist what type of shower shoe would be best for you.

- DO NOT wear plastic flip flops or narrow toed shoes.

Chapter 60

Nail Care And Health

Importance Of Hygiene

Hygiene refers to behaviors that can improve cleanliness and lead to good health, such as frequent hand washing, face washing, and bathing with soap and water. In many areas of the world, practicing personal hygiene etiquette is difficult due to lack of clean water and soap. Many diseases can be spread if the hands, face, or body are not washed appropriately at key times.

- It is estimated that washing hands with soap and water could reduce diarrheal disease-associated deaths by up to 50 percent.

- A large percentage of foodborne disease outbreaks are spread by contaminated hands. Appropriate hand washing practices can reduce the risk of foodborne illness and other infections.

Keeping Hands Clean

Keeping hands clean through improved hand hygiene is one of the most important steps we can take to avoid getting sick and spreading germs to others. Many and conditions are spread by not washing hands with soap and clean, running water. If clean, running water is not accessible, as is common in many parts of the world, use soap and available water. If soap and water are unavailable, use an alcohol-based hand sanitizer that contains at least 60 percent alcohol to clean hands.

About This Chapter: This chapter includes text excerpted from "Water, Sanitation & Environmentally-Related Hygiene," Centers for Disease Control and Prevention (CDC), July 26, 2016.

When Should You Wash Your Hands?

- Before, during, and after preparing food

- Before eating food

- Before and after caring for someone who is sick

- Before and after treating a cut or wound

- After using the toilet

- After changing diapers or cleaning up a child who has used the toilet

- After blowing your nose, coughing, or sneezing

- After touching an animal, animal feed, or animal waste

- After handling pet food or pet treats

- After touching garbage

How Should You Wash Your Hands?

- **Wet** your hands with clean, running water (warm or cold), turn off the tap, and apply soap.

- **Lather** your hands by rubbing them together with the soap. Be sure to lather the backs of your hands, between your fingers, and under your nails.

- **Scrub** your hands for at least 20 seconds. Need a timer? Hum the "Happy Birthday" song from beginning to end twice.

- **Rinse** your hands well under clean, running water.

- **Dry** your hands using a clean towel or air dry them.

What Should You Do If You Don't Have Soap And Clean, Running Water?

Washing hands with soap and water is the best way to reduce the number of germs on them in most situations. If soap and water are not available, use an alcohol-based hand sanitizer that contains at least 60 percent alcohol. Alcohol-based hand sanitizers can quickly reduce the number of germs on hands in some situations, but sanitizers do not eliminate all types of germs and might not remove harmful chemicals.

Hand sanitizers are not as effective when hands are visibly dirty or greasy.

How Do You Use Hand Sanitizers?

- Apply the product to the palm of one hand (read the label to learn the correct amount).

- Rub your hands together.

- Rub the product over all surfaces of your hands and fingers until your hands are dry.

Nail Hygiene

Appropriate hand hygiene includes diligently cleaning and trimming fingernails, which may harbor dirt and germs and can contribute to the spread of some infections, such as pinworms. Fingernails should be kept short, and the undersides should be cleaned frequently with soap and water. Because of their length, longer fingernails can harbor more dirt and bacteria than short nails, thus potentially contributing to the spread of infection.

Before clipping or grooming nails, all equipment (for example, nail clippers and files) should be properly cleaned. Sterilizing equipment before use is especially important when nail tools are shared among a number of people, as is common in commercial nail salons.

Infections of the fingernails or toenails are often characterized by swelling of the surrounding skin, pain in the surrounding area, or thickening of the nail. In some cases, these infections may be serious and need to be treated by a physician.

To help prevent the spread of germs and nail infections:

- Keep nails short and trim them often.

- Scrub the underside of nails with soap and water (or a nail brush) every time you wash your hands.

- Clean any nail grooming tools before use.

- In commercial settings such as nail salons, sterilize nail grooming tools before use.

- Avoid biting or chewing nails.

- Avoid cutting cuticles, as they act as barriers to prevent infection.

- Never rip or bite a hangnail. Instead, clip it with a clean, sanitized nail trimmer.

Part Seven
If You Need More Information

Chapter 61
Resources For Skin Information

Agricultural Research Service (ARS)
U.S. Department of Agriculture (USDA)
1400 Independence Ave. S.W.
Washington DC, 20250
Phone: 202-720-3656
Fax: 202-720-5427
Website: www.ars.usda.gov/docs/headquarters-information

American Academy of Dermatology (AAD)
P.O. Box 4014
Schaumburg, IL 60168-4014
Toll-Free: 866-503-SKIN (866-503-7546)
Phone: 847-240-1280
Fax: 847-240-1859
Website: www.aad.org/contact-us
E-mail: mrc@aad.org

American Academy of Facial Plastic and Reconstructive Surgery (AAFPRS)
310 S. Henry St.
Alexandria, VA 22314
Phone: 703-299-9291
Fax: 703-299-8898
Website: www.aafprs.org/academy/contactus
E-mail: info@aafprs.org

About This Chapter: Resources in this chapter were compiled from several sources deemed reliable; all contact information was verified and updated in August 2017.

American Academy of Family Physicians (AAFP)

11400 Tomahawk Creek Pkwy
Leawood, KS 66211-2680
Toll-Free: 800-274-2237
Phone: 913-906-6000
Fax: 913-906-6075
Website: www.nf.aafp.org/myacademy/contactus
E-mail: aafp@aafp.org

American Academy of Pediatrics (AAP)

141 N.W. Point Blvd.
Elk Grove Village, IL 60007-1098
Phone: 800-433-9016
Fax: 847-434-8000
Website: www.aap.org/en-us/Pages/Contact.aspx

American Lyme Disease Foundation (ALDF)

P.O. Box 466
Lyme, CT 06371
Website: www.aldf.com/#contact
E-mail: questions@aldf.com

American Osteopathic College of Dermatology (AOCD)

2902 N. Baltimore St.
P.O. Box 7525
Kirksville, MO 63501
Toll-Free: 800-449-2623
Phone: 660-665-2184
Fax: 660-627-2623
Website: www.aocd.org/?page=Contact

American Skin Association (ASA)

335 Madison Ave.
22nd Fl.
New York, NY 10017
Toll-Free: 800-499-SKIN (800-499-7546)
Phone: 212-889-4858
Fax: 212-889-4959
Website: www.americanskin.org/contact
E-mail: info@americanskin.org

American Society for Dermatological Surgery (ASDS)

5550 Meadowbrook Dr.
Ste. 120
Rolling Meadows, IL 60008
Phone: 847-956-0900
Fax: 847-956-0999
Website: www.asds.net

American Society of Plastic Surgeons (ASPS)

The Plastic Surgery Foundation
444 E. Algonquin Rd.
Arlington Heights, IL 60005
Toll-Free: 800-514-5058
Phone: 847-228-9900
Website: www.plasticsurgery.org/about-asps/contact-us

Asthma and Allergy Foundation of America (AAFA)

8201 Corporate Dr.
Ste. 1000
Landover, MD 20785
Toll-Free: 800-7-ASTHMA (800-727-8462)
Fax: 202-466-8940
Website: www.aafa.org/page/asthma-allergy-education-programs-teach-patients.aspx
E-mail: Info@aafa.org

Center for Young Women's Health (CYWH)

333 Longwood Ave.
5th Fl.
Boston, MA 02115
Phone: 617-355-2994
Fax: 617-730-0186
Website: www.youngwomenshealth.org/contact-us
E-mail: cywh@childrens.harvard.edu

Centers for Disease Control and Prevention (CDC)

1600 Clifton Rd.
Atlanta, GA 30329-4027
Toll-Free: 800-CDC-INFO (800-232-4636)
TTY: 888-232-6348
Website: www.cdc.gov

Cleveland Clinic Foundation
9500 Euclid Ave.
Cleveland, OH 44195
Toll-Free: 800-223-2273
Phone: 216-444-2200
TTY: 216-444-0261
Website: www.my.clevelandclinic.org

Federal Trade Commission (FTC)
600 Pennsylvania Ave. N.W.
Washington, DC 20580
Phone: 202-326-2222
Website: www.ftc.gov/contact

Genetic and Rare Diseases Information Center (GARD)
National Center for Advancing Translational Sciences (NCATS)
P.O. Box 8126
Gaithersburg, MD 20898-8126
Toll-Free: 888-205-2311
Website: www.rarediseases.info.nih.gov

Hampton University Skin of Color Research Institute (HUSCRI)
P.O. Box 6035
Hampton, VA 23668
Phone: 757-727-5885
Website: www.huscri.hamptonu.edu/contact
E-mail: info@huscri.org

Health Resources and Services Administration (HRSA)
5600 Fishers Ln.
Rockville, MD 20857
Toll-Free: 877-464-4772
Phone: 301-443-3376
TTY: 877-897-9910
Website: www.hrsa.gov/about/contact

International Hyperhidrosis Society (IHHS)
2560 Township Rd.
Ste. B
Quakertown, PA 18951
Phone: 610-346-6008
Fax: 610-346-6004
Website: www.sweathelp.org
E-mail: info@sweathelp.org

Louisiana State University (LSU) School of Veterinary Medicine
Skip Bertman Dr.
Baton Rouge, LA 70803
Phone: 225-578-9900
Fax: 225-578-9916
Website: www.lsu.edu/vetmed/pbs/contact_us.php
E-mail: vetmed@lsu.edu

Lupus Foundation of America (LFA)
2121 K St. N.W., Ste. 200
Washington, DC 20037
Toll-Free: 800-558-0121
Phone: 202-349-1155
Fax: 202-349-1156
Website: www.lupus.org/about/contact-us
E-mail: info@lupus.org

National Alopecia Areata Foundation (NAAF)
65 Mitchell Blvd.
Ste. 200-B
San Rafael, CA 94903
Phone: 415-472-3780
Fax: 415-480-1800
Website: www.naaf.org/contact
E-mail: info@naaf.org

National Cancer Institute (NCI)
9609 Medical Center Dr.
BG 9609 MSC 9760
Bethesda, MD 20892-9760
Toll-Free: 800-4-CANCER (800-422-6237)
Website: www.cancer.gov/contact

National Eczema Association (NEA)

4460 Redwood Hwy
Ste. 16-D
San Rafael, CA 94903
Toll-Free: 800-818-7546
Phone: 415-499-3474
Website: www.nationaleczema.org/contact
E-mail: info@nationaleczema.org

National Institute of Allergy and Infectious Diseases (NIAID)

Office of Communications and Government Relations
5601 Fishers Ln.
MSC 9806
Bethesda, MD 20892-9806
Toll-Free: 866-284-4107
Phone: 301-496-5717
TDD: 800-877-8339
Fax: 301-402-3573
Website: www.niaid.nih.gov/global/contact-us
E-mail: ocpostoffice@niaid.nih.gov

National Institute of Arthritis and Musculoskeletal and Skin Diseases (NIAMS)

Information Clearinghouse
1 AMS Cir.
Bethesda, MD 20892-3675
Toll-Free: 877-22-NIAMS (877-226-4267)
Phone: 301-495-4484
TTY: 301-565-2966
Fax: 301-718-6366
Website: www.niams.nih.gov/About_Us/Contact_Us/default.asp
E-mail: NIAMSinfo@mail.nih.gov

National Institute of General Medical Sciences (NIGMS)

45 Center Dr.
MSC 6200
Bethesda, MD 20892-6200
Phone: 301-496-7301
Website: www.nigms.nih.gov/Pages/ContactUs.aspx
E-mail: info@nigms.nih.gov

National Psoriasis Foundation (NPF)

6600 S.W. 92nd Ave.
Ste. 300
Portland, OR 97223-7195
Toll-Free: 800-723-9166
Phone: 503-244-7404
Fax: 503-245-0626
Website: www.psoriasis.org/about-us/contact
E-mail: getinfo@psoriasis.org

National Rosacea Society (NRS)

196 James St.
Barrington, IL 60010
Toll-Free: 888-NO-BLUSH (888-662-5874)
Website: www.rosacea.org
E-mail: rosaceas@aol.com

New Zealand Dermatological Society Incorporated (NZDSI)

P.O. Box 4431
Palmerston N.
Manawatu, NY 4442
Phone: 06-357-1466
Fax: 06-357-1426
Website: www.nzdsi.org/Contact.aspx
E-mail: sue@spconferences.co.nz

Office on Women's Health (OWH)

U.S. Department of Health and Human Services (HHS)
200 Independence Ave. S.W.
Rm. 712E
Washington, DC 20201
Toll-Free: 800-994-9662
Phone: 202-690-7650
Fax: 202-205-2631
Website: www.womenshealth.gov/contact-us

Scleroderma Foundation (SF)

300 Rosewood Dr.
Ste. 105
Danvers, MA 01923
Toll-Free: 800-722-HOPE (800-722-4673)
Phone: 978-463-5843
Fax: 978-777-1313
Website: www.scleroderma.org/site/PageServer?pagename=about_contact#.WZFNTd8xDrc
E-mail: sfinfo@scleroderma.org

The Skin Cancer Foundation (SCF)

149 Madison Ave.
Ste. 901
New York, NY 10016
Phone: 212-725-5176
Website: www.skincancer.org/contact-us

The Trichotillomania Learning Center (TLC) Foundation

716 Soquel Ave.
Ste. A
Santa Cruz, CA 95062
Phone: 831-457-1004
Fax: 831-427-5541
Website: www.bfrb.org/discover-your-foundation/contact-us
E-mail: info@bfrb.org

U.S. Food and Drug Administration (FDA)

10903 New Hampshire Ave.
Silver Spring, MD 20993
Toll-Free: 888-INFO-FDA (888-463-6332)
Website: www.fda.gov

U.S. National Library of Medicine (NLM)

8600 Rockville Pike
Bethesda, MD 20894
Toll-Free: 888-FIND-NLM (888-346-3656)
Phone: 301-594-5983
Fax: 301-402-1384
Website: www.nlm.nih.gov/about/index.html
E-mail: custserv@nlm.nih.gov

Vitiligo Support International (VSI)

P.O. Box 3565
Lynchburg, VA 24503
Phone: 434-326-5380
Website: www.vitiligosupport.org/contact.cfm

Women's Dermatologic Society (WDS)

555 E. Wells St.
Ste. 1100
Milwaukee, WI 53202
Toll-Free: 877-WDS-ROSE (877-937-7673)
Fax: 414-272-6070
Website: www.womensderm.org/about-wds/staff
E-mail: wds@womensderm.org

Index

Index

Page numbers that appear in *Italics* refer to tables or illustrations. Page numbers that have a small 'n' after the page number refer to citation information shown as Notes. Page numbers that appear in **Bold** refer to information contained in boxes within the chapters.

A

contact dermatitis, postinflammatory
 hyperpigmentation 16
contracture scars, defined 238
contusion, bruises 234
corns
  described 268
  footcare 327
"Corns And Calluses" (NIH) 267n
corticosteroids
  acne 36
  atopic dermatitis 145
  hives 222
  keloids 165
  lupus 169
  pityriasis rosea 205
  psoriasis 199
  Sutton disease 2 **74**
  vitiligo 226
cosmetics
  acne **27**
  atopic dermatitis **145**
  pruritus 194
  rosacea 207
  tanning **299**
  tips 285
  vitiligo 227
"Cosmetics Safety Q&A: Shelf Life" (FDA) 285n
"Cosmetics: Tips For Women" (FDA) 285n
crusted scabies, described 109
cryosurgery
  scars 238
  skin cancer 179
cuticle, skin picking 271
cuts, treatment 233
cystic acne, treatment 35
cysts, described 135
"Cysts: Epidermoid, Pilonidal, And Lipoma"
 (Omnigraphics) 135n

D

dandruff, described 10
"Dandruff, Cradle Cap, And Other Scalp Conditions"
 (NIH) 3n
deer tick, Lyme disease 67, 255
DEET
  insect repellents 256
  Lyme disease 69
depigmentation, vitiligo 223

depilatories, described 322
depression
  acne 27, 49
  hyperhidrosis 160
  interferon 94
  pruritus 191
  psoriasis 198
  vitiligo 226
dermabrasion
  acne scars 37, **164**, 239
  defined 179
  stretch marks 133
dermatitis
  dandruff 10
  giant congenital melanocytic nevus 130
  see also atopic dermatitis; cercarial dermatitis;
   pseudomonas dermatitis
dermatologist
  acne treatment 28, 33
  actinic keratoses 307
  atopic dermatitis 144
  epidermolysis bullosa 151
  mole changes 190
  rosacea 16, 208
  scleroderma 214
  skin picking 272
  tattoo removal 312
dermis
  depicted *4*
  epidermolysis bullosa 150
  melanoma skin cancer 182
  second-degree burns 241
  skin anatomy 6
DHA *see* dihydroxyacetone
diabetes
  blisters 268
  fungal nail infection 120
  hyperhidrosis 159
  nail discoloration 9
  necrotizing fasciitis 59
  polycystic ovary syndrome 47
  pruritus 191
  waxing 322
dihydroxyacetone (DHA), tanning sprays 301
dog bites, overview 247–50
drug-induced lupus, defined **170**
Drysol, hyperhidrosis 160
dust mite allergy
  atopic dermatitis 146
  hives 222